W9-CFL-086

PRAISE FOR *The Other Side of Desire*

"Unsettling but riveting. . . . On one level, this book has all the elements of a top-rated HBO series—provocatively graphic sex, humorous dialogue, and moral ambiguity. But what makes it so powerful is that it's as much about desire and what's normal as it is an exploration of why we are the way we are, whether we like it or not."   —*New York Times Book Review*

"What's remarkable about Bergner's book is not the way these tales shock or confound or titillate (though they do those things sometimes), but how sympathetic their plights and hungers become. Bergner, whose previous books include *God of the Rodeo*, about convicts in Louisiana's Angola prison, is a keen storyteller but above all a humane one, and in his hands, these characters do not seem like freaks so much as shadows of ourselves."   —*Salon.com*

"Bergner is the kind of author who is able to delve deeply into the darkest and most forbidden realms of the human psyche and behavior. By deftly blending curiosity and compassion in *The Other Side of Desire*, Bergner shows that, if he had not chosen a career as a journalist, he would have made an exceptionally good psychotherapist."   —*San Francisco Chronicle*

"Fully immersed in his subjects, Bergner elicits candor while keeping an ear out for those details that make subjects come to life. . . . Sensationalism would be cheap and easy. Bergner instead extends his characters generosity, seeking explanations rather than casting judgment. His is a meaningful reflection on desire, a need shared by nearly all."
                      —*Time Out New York*

"Bergner does what science cannot: He illuminates peculiar longings. His method is at first descriptive and finally poetic. . . . Given the limitations of science, resonant journalism may be the best way to approach paraphilia, and Bergner's book has a musical quality."　　—Slate.com

"With a minimum of psychobabble and a maximum of tight-focus, unsentimental, unsqueamish reporting, Mr. Bergner tells the story of four people with 'abnormal' sex lives. . . . The author's cool, authoritative tone and openhearted acceptance of what he's exposing wash away all taint of kinky, vicarious thrill. It's enough to make you think that in this case, good reporting isn't just morally neutral. It spreads the love."
　　　　　　　　　　　　　　　　　　—*New York Observer*

"Bergner does an excellent job of humanizing his subjects. Passion is as instinctual as thirst or the need to sleep. While most of us may live on this side of desire, Bergner's book helps us begin to understand the other side, and what it is like to live with the torture of helplessly desiring what society deems unacceptable."　　　　　　　—*Richmond Times-Dispatch*

"In what could have been the worst kind of leering anthropology, Bergner instead finds compassion, sympathy, and even commonality. He calls the stories in the book 'autobiographical,' and the book makes clear that its subjects will provide all of us with convex mirrors reflecting our own sexual desires and practices."　　　　　　　　　　　—Nerve.com

"The book's strength lies in its attentive, carefully controlled tone. . . . Bergner does ask us to try to understand people who often feel like the Hunchback of Notre Dame or are driven to suicide, and to admire some of them for finding a harmless way to live outside the norm. His goal is empathy. He gives depth and shadow to his subjects' longing, never mocking, oversimplifying, or vilifying." —*Washington Post Book World*

"In this fascinating book, Bergner, with a novelist's eye but a reporter's grit, examines amputee devotees and S&M fanatics without resorting to sensationalism." —*Metro New York*

"Girded with scientific data about the nature of sexual identity, *The Other Side of Desire* is a foray into extreme passion, in quest of the human soul." —*O, The Oprah Magazine*

"Bergner investigates how 'we become who we are sexually, whether our lusts are common or improbable.' The book's combination of titillation, shock value, and documentary evokes a set of page-turning conundrums." —*Publishers Weekly* (starred review)

"In carefully etched prose, Bergner unpacks the tightly twisted roots of desire, power seeking, self-hatred, and theatricality that motivate his four pseudonymous subjects. . . . Compassionate wisdom about dark needs." —*Kirkus Reviews*

"In a culture that pays clamorous lip service to the ideal of tolerance, Daniel Bergner's *The Other Side of Desire* is that rare instance of the real thing. The author levels a curious yet compassionate gaze at his subjects, who grapple with the way desire disfigures and exalts. In their struggles to accept themselves for wanting what they want, they are desperate, and often, heroic figures." —Will Blythe, author of *To Hate Like This Is to Be Happy Forever*

ALSO BY DANIEL BERGNER

FICTION

Moments of Favor

NONFICTION

God of the Rodeo:
*The Quest for Redemption in
Louisiana's Angola Prison*

In the Land of Magic Soldiers:
*A Story of White and Black in
West Africa*

THE OTHER
SIDE OF
DESIRE

FOUR JOURNEYS

INTO THE

FAR REALMS OF

LUST AND LONGING

$\mathcal{D}$ANIEL $\mathcal{B}$ERGNER

ecco

An Imprint of HarperCollinsPublishers

HarperCollins books may be purchased for educational, business, or sales promotional use. For information, please e-mail the Speical Markets Department at SPsales@harpercollins.com.

Part of "The Water's Edge" originally appeared in the *New York Times Magazine* on January 23, 2005.

A hardcover edition of this book was published in 2009 by Ecco, an imprint of HarperCollins Publishers.

FIRST ECCO PAPERBACK EDITION PUBLISHED 2010.

Designed by Lucy Albanese and Jessica Shatan Heslin

Library of Congress Cataloging-in-Publication Data

Bergner, Dan (Daniel)
The Other Side of Desire : four journeys into the far realms of lust and longing / Daniel Bergner. — 1st ed.
    p. cm.
1. Paraphilias—Case studies. 2. Compulsive behavior—Case studies. I. Title.
HQ71.B356 2008
306.77--dc22
2007050699
ISBN 978-0-06-088557-1

15 16 17 18 19 ID/RRD   10 9 8 7 6 5

CONTENTS

INTRODUCTION

"What," the people I write about often ask, "are you doing here with me?" I heard the question in Angola Prison, Louisiana's maximum security penitentiary, where I followed the lives of men sentenced to stay locked up until their deaths, with no chance of parole. I heard it in Sierra Leone, in West Africa, where I attached myself to missionaries and mercenaries and child soldiers amid the most brutal war in recent memory. And I heard it as I sought the stories—of eros, obsession, anarchy, love—that fill *The Other Side of Desire*.

It was four years ago that I entered the worlds of the people whose lives form the spine of this book. There was an advertising executive who celebrated the most conventional kind of female beauty in the billboards he created, who felt no attraction to the models he cast, and who was drawn erotically, inescapably, to amputees; there was a clothing designer and rare female sadist who searched for transcendent connection with those she wounded and enslaved; there was a traveling salesman and devoted husband whose fetish brought him extreme ecstasy and crippling abasement; and there was a band leader transfixed by his young stepdaughter.

How do we come to have the particular desires that drive us, how do we become who we are sexually, whether our lusts are common or improbable? How much are we born with and how much do we learn from all that surrounds us, how much can we change and how much is locked unreachably, permanently within? These questions were part of what pulled me toward my four central characters—and toward a set of scientists immersed in studying eros. And then there was the question of how we live with our longings. A speech therapist for stroke victims, a tiny woman with a doll's round face, with black button eyes and a slender, fragile nose, told me that if a dominant lover whispered in her ear in the right way, she could reach orgasm without touch. She wanted to be harmed. But she was tortured by her desire— she was an Orthodox Jew; her grandparents had been slaughtered in the Holocaust; and she couldn't reconcile the cravings of eros with the cruelty her family had suffered. What do we do with the desires we cannot bear, the desires we or the society around us strain to restrict or strangle, whether the wanting is unusual or as typical as the yearning for new lovers that can turn otherwise happy marriages into arrangements that sometimes feel as agonizing as actual imprisonment? And what is the relationship between the physical and the transcendent, between the surfaces of the body and the wish to melt the bounds of self, between the forces of lust and our striving for love?

Some in these stories feared they would be shunned if their private selves were known—I have changed some names and a very few identifying details in order to protect them. As for the question they asked, my answer is, always, this: I am here with you, at the far edges of experience, in the hope that your stories illuminate truths shared by all of us.

PART I

The Phantom of the Opera

JACOB MILLER LOVED TORONTO. HE THOUGHT OF it every day. He was American, and lived in a snowy American city, but a Canadian flag, with its broad bars of red and its red maple leaf, hung in his home office. A printout of the flag, on a sheet of computer paper, was taped to the wall between his kitchen and dining room. Pasted to the rear window of his car, a flag decal hinted at his love. When he dressed casually in wintertime, he favored a letterman's-style jacket. The leaf, big and bright, adorned the back.

If he'd won the lottery, he would have retired and moved to Toronto. If he could have designed his own world, that city would have occupied his entire planet. "When we had our son, I wanted what I call a T-R name," he said, laughing at himself. "Tristan. Troy. Trice. I didn't tell my wife why. I didn't tell her, 'Because it would remind me of Toronto.' She said, 'I'm not naming him Tristan, kids are going to make fun of him. I'm not naming him Troy.' She said, 'What kind of name is Trice?'"

Toronto was a realm where everyone was accepted. On Yonge Street, during a visit in his twenties, twenty years in the past, he'd seen the kids in their punk gear, the parents pushing strollers, the beggars with their cups, the prostitutes in their spandex, the gays hand in hand, all intermixed, passing each other on the sidewalk, tolerating each other, yes, but more than that, seeming tacitly to welcome each other. He'd filled the beggars' cups. Toronto, he felt, was a place even for monsters, a city for men such as himself.

JACOB owned a tidy wooden house not far from downtown in the city where he'd grown up. In the living room, plants cascaded from the mantelpiece; a flat-screen TV was mounted above the greenery. The furniture was soft and stylish. A small white-haired dog trotted across the carpet. The ashes of another, a terrier-beagle he still mourned a decade after its death, sat on a shelf in a box painted gold.

In the driveway, in the months when it wasn't covered in snow, he played basketball with his eight-year-old son, his only child. Ben was dark-haired, frail. They shot at a portable hoop Jacob had bought, lowered to a height the boy could manage. Jacob himself had never been much for sports, but Ben had lately taught him to play Pig. "It's easy, Pop!" he'd cried out. "It's easy!" So they shot and talked, shot and talked. Ben had suffered a stroke during his fifth month in the womb and had cerebral palsy. In the winter months, Jacob was teaching him to ski.

He'd been married to Ben's mother for sixteen years. He'd thought her beautiful when they met; he thought her beautiful now. "I've had men say to me, 'You're a lucky guy.'" She had a profusion of black hair and smooth olive skin and large dark eyes. She was petite and full-breasted. She'd come from a small town, and he took her, on their first date, to a restaurant she saw as dazzling. Over a dinner much more expensive than she was used to, he learned about her job for an airline, at a ticket counter, which allowed her to fly for free. This struck him as glamorous. And he told her about his success as a sales-man. "This gorgeous woman," he remembered. "She put me on a pedestal, and I put her on a pedestal."

He still felt they were wonderfully matched. "We're home-body people," he said, listing the things they loved to do to-gether: sit on the porch and watch Ben ride his bicycle or his electric scooter; go to craft shows and collect southwestern ceramics decorated with a flute-playing figure called Koko-pelli. After sixteen years, they still called each other from work three or four times a day.

Jacob had put together this life of comfort and love despite at least two relevant obstacles. One was a learning disability so extreme that, in his mid-forties, he could read sentences and calculate numbers no better than most fourth-graders. He'd been given special glasses as a child, with cardboard frames and one green and one red lens. For much of each school day, he'd been made to wear this clownish gear.

The remedy hadn't worked; the only way he'd kept up at all was that classmates read his assignments into a reel-to-reel, and at night he lay in bed, listening. When Jacob was in his late thirties, the head psychiatrist at the hospital of Johns Hopkins University had used him to instruct his stu-dents. With Jacob's consent, the psychiatrist had placed him within a U of sixty pupils, and asked him to imagine hav-ing seventeen apples and giving away five—how many would he have left? Jacob couldn't answer. There were more ques-tions like it, and a simple paragraph he stumbled through and couldn't comprehend. Then, after the stymied gasps of the psychiatrists-in-training, the head made his point about people's ability to overcome. For Jacob was prosperous, thriving in his job. He kept his customers, across a vast swath of territory along the Great Lakes, unfailingly supplied in the goods he handled, and he supervised a team of junior salespeople. Painstakingly, he managed never to jumble his accounts. He could have carried out his business almost entirely by phone and the Internet, but, always anxious that no one should be unhappy with him, he drove for hours and hours each day to present himself in person, a slightly short, husky man, neatly dressed in a jacket and turtleneck or tie— just to shake hands and chat for a few minutes, just to ask his customers if they had any complaints and reassure them that he would make all adjustments.

The second obstacle had to do with sex.

Jacob was, in psychiatric terms, a paraphiliac, the word being an amalgam of two ancient roots, *para* meaning "alongside" or "beyond" and *philia* meaning "love." The focus of his love, the focus of his desire, fell outside the normal zones. He was drawn to women's feet. The feet were the breasts, the legs, the buttocks, the genitals. He wanted, dizzyingly, to touch them, hold them, gaze upon them, lick them, suck them, press his cock against them, slide his cock across them, have a woman position her feet together—the sides of the paired arches forming a kind of footcunt—so he could fuck them.

I should make two things clear about terminology. First, some among the psychiatric experts on sex—the sexologists, as the descendants of Kinsey are called—would have insisted that Jacob wasn't a paraphiliac, that, rather, he *had* a paraphilia, the difference being one of identity versus affliction. Either he was defined by the paraphilia or it was something far from his center, something visited upon him, locked to him, asserting itself dictatorially within him, but defining him no more than anyone can be defined by a disease.

Second, Jacob would never have used a word like "fuck," let alone "cunt." He was a somewhat shy and very decorous man. He said "intercourse" if he had to say anything at all.

Decorous and dizzy, he felt mortified by his longing. A strange and nearly complete substitution had occurred, leaving him, he felt, infinitely different from other men. He cared about faces, and a woman's figure wasn't irrelevant. When he spoke about his wife's beauty, he meant what other men do. But without the feet there was no palpable desire. When he recalled his first date with his wife, he couldn't remember what she'd been wearing in the usual sense. It seemed that from the ankles up all had been attractive but vague. Yet he recalled, vividly, her open-toed shoes with modest heels and a beige leather strap crossing just above the base of her toes.

His erotic distortion made him hideous in his eyes. He clung to the concept of affliction but plummeted into the vortex of identity. Yet there were psychiatrists and psychologists, clinicians and researchers, who believed that he had a gift. For intensity, they told me, there was no comparison between the experience of someone like Jacob and the experience of those they termed "the normophilic." For sheer driven need, for keen and exalted erotic hunger, for the loss of consciousness that typical desire and typical sex may never provide or may offer only at the instant of orgasm and even then not quite completely despite the brain's dimness and the involuntary cries, for true negation of control and obliteration of self, Jacob had been granted something superior. He owned the chance for ecstasy.

• • •

NEXT to the second-grade classroom of Jacob's childhood was a cubby area where the kids had tugged off their rubber snow boots; sometimes their socks slipped off in the process. It was his earliest memory of the yearning which, as a child, he'd had no reason to think strange. The closest he came to touching, back then, was with a boy who played at his house. For a few years it was boys' feet that transfixed him; with puberty the effect switched over to girls. One afternoon he scurried frantically to set something, anything, high in his closet while the boy was out of the room. He tossed a ball up onto a shelf, then told his friend he couldn't reach it. The boy said he would try. Jacob told him to take off his shoes and to put his foot in the stirrup formed by his hands.

Jacob recognized his difference when, seeing the pictures of naked women that stirred other boys, he felt nothing. A retreat from the world, an isolation that had begun with the red and green lenses, deepened. His grandmother's house had always been his refuge. When the days of clownish headgear grew unbearable, he sometimes sprang out of his chair and out of the classroom, crashed out the school's side doors, and staggered through the snow on the school's sloping field, making it to the road and running up the long hill to her home. She was somewhat strange herself, an old woman who drove a red Cadillac but kept her house frigid and sat in the dark to cut her bills, and she guarded him fiercely, refusing to send him back to school despite his parents' pleas.

And later, when he was in his teens, she called him constantly to her house to make repairs. She pointed out a crack in the plaster of her ceiling, directed him to get her ladder, and handed him a roll of scotch tape. Crazy though he felt she was, he taped the fissure as he was told. "No one could have fixed that ceiling like you!" she exclaimed. It was the same with installing storm windows every autumn: "No one can put up storm windows like you!" And cutting her grass: "You're the only one who can mow that lawn!"

The first girl he fell in love with walked into his life with her grandmother. He was working in a sporting goods store, having dropped out of college because every assignment was beyond him. Standing beside her grandmother, the girl asked to try on a pair of Nike Cortez. It was the style he had on, his favorite sneaker: low and simple and streamlined, with a thin, serrated sole that resembled a long row of tiny teeth. And she wanted the very color scheme he was wearing: white with a red Nike swoosh. He didn't have a fetish for shoes in themselves, but her choice seemed to him a sign. He was a romantic man, a sentimental man. A hint of destiny seemed to lie in their taste in sneakers.

He learned, too, the size and width of her feet. He'd always liked large feet; just to hear the words "size eight" or "size nine" could make him hard. Hers were a seven and a half, but wide. He sat on the salesman's low stool; she placed her feet, one after the other, on the inclined platform between his legs. He slid the heels over her white sweat socks, tightened and tied the laces. She paced around, declared that they fit, tried on other styles, returned to her original choice, then lingered, chatting, apologizing: "I know you have to get going." Her pale, pretty, tentative face spoke to him of tenderness, empathy. He told her he didn't have to go at all, and as the conversation veered she mentioned that she lived with her grandmother.

"I live with *my* grandmother." He had recently moved into her frigid, comforting house.

"Get out!"

"I do, I do! I'm telling you the truth!" But when at last she left with her sneakers—her name was Sara—he was sure he would never see her again.

He remembered: "Her grandmother and her were joined at the hip, exactly like my grandmother and I were. Her grandmother was petite, the same as mine. And she was extremely frugal, just like mine."

He didn't yet know these details when he spotted her a week later in the store, again with the old woman, and heard himself, witless: "You're back."

"I came back to see you."

He turned right away to the woman, asking for their phone number, then blurted out an invitation to both of them, wondering if he could take them to dinner. They said he should come to their house instead. His first date with Sara—she was fifteen, he was twenty-one—was a kind of threesome. The grandmother cooked meat and mashed potatoes while he sat with the granddaughter in a porch room, her feet bare. They joked about their width. "Platypus feet," he said, "you have platypus feet," the two of them laughing, giggling. Her toes formed a perfect staircase, each one, from big toe to pinkie, successively smaller, defining a gentle descent.

When her grandmother called them in to eat he raced up and down his mind's corridors, peering into corners, searching for something to distract him from his desire, something to diminish it. The old woman's voice, like a glancing eye on the brink of noticing his perversion, had pierced his brain. He could find no distraction. His brain was a void, except for the one thing he wanted to escape.

But at the table he managed to function, and afterward, as he and Sara watched TV, she placed her feet on an ottoman. In her toes and tendons and arches and heels was concentrated all the combined power of all the more common erotic parts upon more common men. The staircase was his ideal, and the platypus-like width made her his version of a swimsuit model, and hesitantly he took her feet, each in turn, in his hands, and while she pretended to focus on the television he began to massage them—delicately, adoringly—as though nothing else existed in the world.

JACOB was Jewish, and when he confided his love to his grandmother she asked about the girl's religion. The answer wasn't the right one. But soon his grandmother, who hated dogs and wanted them nowhere near, came to love the mutt— the terrier-beagle whose ashes now rested on his living room mantel—that he and Sara bought together after spotting it in a pet shop cage during a stroll at a mall. By that point he had moved into his own apartment, and one morning his grandmother phoned, demanding that he come over right away. She'd seen a mouse and declared herself scared to death. "Bring the *hunt*!" she ordered, using the Yiddish word for dog.

"His name is Max," Jacob said.

"Just bring the *hunt*!"

He did, the mouse disappeared, and from then on she wanted the dog to visit all the time and deemed both Jacob and Sara heroes for owning it: "No one can scare mice like that *hunt*!"

Sara's grandmother was grateful for the stability he offered; Sara's high school friends struck her as wild. Her grandmother wanted only to know that he would be a gentleman, that he and Sara weren't doing anything they shouldn't during their hours in the TV room after the meals she prepared. He gave her his word, and for three years he kept it. His palms and fingers and lips and tongue traveled from her feet to her breasts and back again, the care of the trip upward masking the urgency of the trip down. Preserving her virginity wasn't a problem for him. He came explosively, in secret, in the bathroom, never confessing his desire. But with all the attention to her body, all the signals he sent surging through her calves and thighs and breasts, chastity became a problem for her. She begged him for sex; he held off until she turned eighteen, then entered her with her feet in his hands or glimpsed in the corners of his eyes or—he needed this at the very least—pictured in his mind.

She was still in high school when she began to talk about marriage. He insisted that they live together first, needing to be sure that all wouldn't unravel. When she started college, she took up with a new set of friends, began smoking marijuana, grew distant from him. "I started to feel like a sugar daddy," he recalled. One day he turned a street corner and saw her hand in hand with someone else. Sara's grandmother was as desolate as he was when they separated. She asked if he wanted to move in with her. For several weeks he ate her dinners, watched her television, slept under her roof.

And more than twenty years later, as I sat in his living room, he asked if I'd like to see Sara's picture, and darted upstairs to slide it from wherever he kept it hidden. It was a small print with the posed and creamy look of a yearbook portrait. Her shoulder-length brown hair was carefully yet simply styled; her pale skin looked flawless to the point of appearing almost blurred; her smile was bright but seemed on the verge of collapse, like the smiles of so many teenage girls when faced with a photographer's scrutiny and the prospect of a yearbook's permanence. I couldn't think of much to say as we gazed at her face together, but he filled the silence. "Not a day goes by when I don't think about her. I had a psychologist once who told me, 'Jacob, there's a lid for every pot.' There's my lid." He struggled to express exactly why, and returned, again and again, to their common love of their grandmothers, as though Sara was linked so strongly to the solace his grandmother had given him growing up that he needed nothing, in addition, besides the rush of attraction—and the perfection of her feet had offered him that. "There's my lid," he said again, then pleaded, "Don't make me cry here."

It wasn't clear with whom he was pleading: I wasn't talking, and the photograph seemed far too inexpressive to elicit tears. Yet he was seeing things I could not see, feeling things he could not communicate. His grandmother had been a woman of ultimate understanding, intuiting his shame and protecting him from the world that inflicted it. The miswiring of his brain had held him back a year in elementary school and made his advancement afterward a matter of sheer mercy, but she had provided a realm where this was irrelevant, and where his ability to scotch-tape a ceiling was a princely virtue. He never told her anything about the second way his brain had betrayed him, about the fact that he wasn't driven at all to place himself inside a vagina but was desperate instead to be between a pair of feet, about the way his brain seemed to have set on the hood of his penis a pair of red-and-green glasses, about the way sex flooded him with self-loathing. He had no reason to think she had gleaned even a hint of it. Yet her acceptance and admiration had always been so unconditional and complete that they could seem to include his secret.

A few times, in the four and a half years he and Sara had been together, as he licked and kneaded her feet yet again, she whispered, teasing, "I think you like my feet better than anything."

"What are you talking about?"

"I think," she breathed, "you've got a problem." But she whispered it sweetly, as though suggesting that she didn't mind, and the flood of self-loathing was drowned in a tide of gratitude.

"Don't make me cry here," he repeated in his living room, and turned, and stepped past the printout of the Canadian flag and up the stairs to return her portrait to its dark, sacred place.

IN winter, Jacob tried not to listen to the weather report. A blizzard might easily bring a foot of snow, or over a foot, or two or three feet in the serious storms. The blizzards came one after another, and he couldn't bear the word. "Imagine if snowfall was measured in breasts and you were the only man with that sick desire," he tried to explain. "If you had to hear the weatherman saying, *breasts, breasts, breasts, breasts, breasts*, and you were the only one who knew. You'd kept it hidden since you were a kid."

With each passing year, through his late twenties and into his thirties, the craving, compounded by the secrecy, grew in strength. "You have to laugh," he said, and did, at himself. "People don't realize it. How many times that word comes up. If you said, 'Jacob, I'm renovating my house, how many square feet do you think the study needs to be?' I'd think, Square feet, I wouldn't mind looking at some square feet."

The winter was difficult, too, because guests at his house thought they should take off their shoes or boots. It was simple courtesy. "'Not in my house,' I'll say. 'We don't do that.'

"'Oh, I don't want to mess up your floor.'

"'Don't worry about it.'

"'But it's no trouble, really. I don't want to track up your carpet.'

"'No, no, please, we'll clean it up, we don't mind, we clean all the time, we'll vacuum the carpet. Please.'"

But late spring was the worst of all, with its sudden sandals and flip-flops, its abrupt emergence of feet that seemed especially bare for being untanned. Once, driving, with the traffic clogged at a construction site, a car came to a stop next to him. The young woman in the passenger seat had her feet up on the dash, and he exploded within seconds, scarcely touching himself. Sometimes he didn't need any contact with his penis at all. He could reach orgasm simply from the feel of feet in his palms or against his tongue, or from the sight of a high arch or a broad instep.

Television besieged him. On a cop show, a tough female detective warned a suspect, "I'm going to stick my size eight where the sun don't shine." It seemed that every movie had a scene with bare feet. Yet sitting in a doctor's office he picked up a magazine that listed Hollywood celebrities according to their best body part. "They had every part but one," he remembered, feeling utterly alone. He understood that the existence of pornographic Web sites catering to his desire could only mean that there were other men like himself, but the others, he was sure, had milder, more passing interests. No other mind was so thoroughly scrambled as his own. "My point," he said, after describing the magazine that hadn't praised the feet of a single movie star, "is that obviously it's not acceptable." He paused, then asked me, "Do you think your wife would accept it?

"I'll be honest with you," he answered himself. "I wouldn't *want* my wife to accept it."

He confided in no one. He conducted surveys. They would begin with a photograph in the sports section, a college or high school girl on a softball field or basketball court; he'd always been taken with the idea of athletic feet. Working from the caption, he would call information for the girl's number. The survey stuck to a script: "Hello, I'm calling from Nike, and we're putting out a new sneaker. We're doing a sixty-second survey today. Would you mind answering a few questions? . . . Do you wear sneakers? . . . Do you play sports? . . . Can you tell me what size you are? . . . Are your feet narrow or wide? . . . Now, if you saw two girls sucking on each other's toes, would you find that disgusting or would you find that funny?" He thanked them politely as soon as he'd come, felt beset by guilt as soon as he'd hung up.

In restaurants, he sometimes knocked a woman's dangled pump from her toes as he edged between tables. When he apologized, the woman would give her reassurance: "Don't worry, it's nothing." But it wasn't nothing. "No matter where you go," he said, "there are people, and people have feet. Unless I lived in a center for amputees. That would be peace."

The ads for massage parlors filled the back pages of the city's alternative magazine, and he'd stared at them countless times, warning himself, "You can't do that, you can't just pay your money and take a girl's body, you can't." But in his late thirties, he found himself in a dimly lit greeting room. Six young women stood in front of him—in stilettos, in lesser heels, in sandals—instructing him to choose. His eyes scanned faces and swooped toward the floor; he picked a woman with toes that formed the staircase of his fantasy.

He followed her along a corridor into a small room of their own. "Okay," she said, turning to face him, "whatever you want."

He didn't answer.

"I'm going to give you a condom."

He stayed silent.

"Is it a blow job you're interested in?"

"No, I'm not interested in that."

"You're not?" Her voice climbed slightly.

"No."

"Well, what interests you then?"

He couldn't speak. She held the condom out toward him a second time.

"We're not going to need that."

Something shifted in her eyes. "You paid me sixty dollars, what are we going to do?"

"Take your shoes off."

"What?"

"Don't worry."

She did as she was told, and stood in her bare feet.

"Now lie back on the bed."

He let down his pants. She asked if she should undress; he whispered that she didn't have to. His hands and mouth had begun.

"You got to be kidding," she said. "You're paying me to do this?"

He couldn't force himself to pull his lips away to answer. But he lifted them away to put his cock where he'd always dreamed of sliding it. The sensation swallowed him, spirited him into unconsciousness.

"I'm going to give you my card," she said, afterward. "Anytime you want to come back, please, you let me know. You're going to be my favorite customer."

THE guilt he felt for renting her body; the humiliation of her words, *You're going to be my favorite customer*; the relentless urge to have her again; the jolt of panic that came with learning, some weeks later, that the place had been raided, that he could have been among the men rounded up—all of this pushed him toward treatment.

He'd been in therapy before, the standard sessions of talking. Nothing had changed, except that he had tried to tell his wife. The therapist had demanded it, saying she could not work with him if he didn't, and so one October night, as they were driving home on an empty highway after a dinner with friends, he forced himself to speak, relieved at least to have his face in darkness and his eyes fixed on the road. But he used general phrases, "I have a sexual problem," "I have a sexual addiction," and his wife started crying, asking only if he'd had an affair. It wasn't an unlikely fear: he avoided sex with her, as he always had, out of dread that he would reveal the hideous need at his core. He assured her he hadn't. He alluded to the Internet, the telephone, barely mentioning the word "feet." Sobbing, she said she didn't understand. He told her he didn't either. He invited her to join him with the therapist, but she refused, didn't talk to Jacob for two days, and when the silence was over it was almost as though, on that desolate October highway, nothing had been said.

Now, after his session with the prostitute, he flew to Baltimore to seek the help of a psychiatrist who, he'd read, was among the greatest experts in the country on sexual disorders. Fred Berlin worked in a vast and grand Victorian house, with a façade of rust-colored bricks and turrets at the corners. It stood on a hill above the harbor. The stoop was high, the outer vestibule was towering and dark, the massive wooden front doors were elaborately carved. There was no sign on any exterior wall of the building, nor on the doors nor below the doorbell, to name what was inside. Once, he'd seen nearly all his patients at his office at the hospital of Johns Hopkins University, and he still taught at Hopkins and did rounds at the hospital (where, after becoming Berlin's patient, Jacob would help the head psychiatrist to instruct his students). But the university, it seemed to Berlin, had grown terribly uncomfortable with his practice—most of which involved not only the aberrant but the criminal—so he had moved his main work away from the campus to this private castle.

Inside, the floorboards had a soft gleam, as did the banisters, which were capped at each landing by an intricate wooden sphere. All was dim and quiet and burnished. But the immense waiting room held plants and small trees with leaves the size of platters; they stretched their anarchic limbs toward each other and over the backs of the plush couches. A glass coffee table was supported not by legs but by part of a contorted tree trunk, aggressively gnarled and adding to the suggestion of encroaching jungle.

There was, too, a seven-foot-high grandfather clock that stood in one corner. Within the glass case the brass pendulum swung along its gentle, unremitting arc, its face bearing the Hopkins seal. It sometimes seemed that this steadiness, this emblem of prestige, tamed the plant life. At other times, when a waiting patient decided to turn on the large television, and to turn the volume up high, the wordless battle between the jungle and the clock felt irrelevant. All was consumed by the human need to drown out one's inner voices with the blaring voices of TV.

The offices Berlin shared with his few partners were furnished with antiques. Stately desks and lush, splendid chairs filled the rooms. He'd done much of the decorating himself, and took pride in the ambience of age and grandeur. But one object didn't fit. A detailed model of a sports stadium, made of wood and metal, sat on a desk in a room used for evaluations—

the stadium of the University of Pittsburgh, where he'd played football during his freshman year on a team that starred a future NFL Hall-of-Famer and that finished the season ranked second in the nation. Berlin had been a bench-sitting line-backer, but the memory of going out for the team, of taking on that challenge four decades ago, still fed his resilience, his determination to be kind toward those whom others would only condemn.

Something of the linebacker lingered in his body, in the barrel-like build, though all had been layered and softened by years. As a sophomore, he'd won a research stipend in psychology, and he never played competitive football again. But the eagerness and energy that impelled him to try out for the team still radiated from his broad shoulders and from the scalp of his round head through his thin, closely cropped hair.

He might have been related to Jacob; they might even have been brothers: both men were short and wide and compressed in the neck, stubby. Both had full cheeks that were beginning to fall toward their crisp shirt collars. Jacob's head, too, was covered minimally in well-trimmed hair; a warm energy emanated from both their skulls. And even their voices shared a slightly high pitch and faint scratchiness.

Yet there were differences that added up to something unmistakable. Berlin's body was more solid, his face more firm. His entire presence held a combination of sensitivity and stubborn, quiescent embattlement, while Jacob's spoke of caring but not an immovable core. It was as though they had been carried together in the same womb, but that some prenatal event, some seemingly insignificant but unequal firing of hormones or brief jarring of the amniotic sac, had routed Jacob's life toward the precarious and Berlin's toward strength.

• • •

BERLIN liked to consider human erotic life from the vantage of a Martian scientist gazing down at Earth. "He would see that a lot of different sexual interests exist within the people who live on this planet. He would note people attracted to adults of the opposite gender and people attracted to adults of the same gender and a percentage of people on Earth attracted to children and people attracted to all sorts of other things and aroused by all sorts of behaviors, but the Martian scientist would simply observe these Earthly desires and define their differences, with no judgment or value attached to them."

He had worked with Jeffrey Dahmer, who'd killed seventeen boys and young men, copulating with and cannibalizing the dead bodies. He had testified at trial that Dahmer was afflicted with necrophilia, that he was nearly incapable of becoming aroused with a living person. Berlin had spent time, too, with Michael Ross, who'd confessed to raping and strangling to death eight girls and young women. After two decades of investigations and trials and appeals, Ross wanted to die. He'd told his lawyers to stop filing briefs and arguing on his behalf, to surrender, and as execution approached Berlin hoped that the prisoner would allow him to visit, to say good-bye, perhaps to be there for him in his last moments.

Ross was, by Berlin's diagnosis, a sexual sadist. "God or nature put sex into each of us," Berlin said, as we sat on the ornate red chairs in one corner of his expansive office. "If we don't eat, we die. If we stop having sex, we perish as a species. We are talking about a powerful, biologically based appetite. And if that drive gets aimed in the wrong direction it still wants to be satisfied. You know, sleep is another biologically based drive—you could promise yourself all you want that you're not going to give in to that craving for sleep, but let me tell you, eventually you're going to. That's the struggle some people are having sexually."

And that was the way he saw even a case so extreme: that here was a man for whom sexual release depended on inflicting terror and torture, a man who had, in effect, restrained himself except for those eight times, those eight acts of primal gratification—such a tiny fraction of the number that most adults seek and find.

"Ultimately," Berlin went on, thinking about the period of the killings, "there was a man in there struggling to do right. He says he tried to talk himself out of leaving the house, fought with himself not to leave, so he wouldn't kill. People want not to believe this. People can't deal with the humanity within a man like Ross. He never wanted to be this kind of person. We can all say, 'Well, he should have turned himself in.' But *people*," Berlin's voice rose as he addressed an invisible outraged throng, "let's take even something as simple as getting a traffic ticket. You don't say to the policeman, 'Oh, and by the way, I do speed frequently.' And you don't turn yourself in for something that will get you executed. What he would tell himself is, 'I'm never going to do it again, and if I turn myself in it doesn't bring back the people who are dead.'"

Berlin's brown eyes glanced abruptly almost straight upward. Then he hunched forward, tight fists held half an inch from his lowered forehead. "I know this all must sound insane to the families of the victims, but to say that Michael Ross is evil just is not accurate, given my knowledge of sexual disorders and the impairment of both cognition and volition. Society can't consider the complexity. You might read about a sexually sadistic serial killer, and the neighbors say, 'Gee, we knew him, we can't believe he's someone who could do that. If you had a flat tire he was going to come over and help you change it.' But the criminal behavior never was a reflection of the personality, the visible aspects of it—it was part of the privacy of the sexual makeup. You and I could sit next to each other, and I don't ask you about your sexuality and you don't ask me about mine, so if the only thing that makes me dangerous is what's driving me sexually, you could be the next-door neighbor, you could be the wife, and never know. I had a patient, a serial rapist, who'd had a girlfriend he wanted to marry. But the urge to engage in coercive sex was so much stronger than the arousal by consenting sex that he would leave the consenting relationship to go out and engage in the coercive. And the girlfriend had no idea until he was arrested."

On death row, with Berlin counseling and encouraging him, Ross had begun injections of Depo Lupron, an anti-androgen. For most patients, at a sufficient dose, the drug cuts the production of testosterone to the degree that desire is severely attenuated; the effect, though reversible if the drug is stopped, is known as chemical castration. Before taking "the medicine," Berlin said, Ross was contrite about his crimes, but there was something robotic about his compunction. "He confessed everything, but he himself described that he knew how he should feel about what he'd done, and that the emotions simply wouldn't well up inside. Intellectually he was sorry, intellectually he felt for the families, but he knew he should be overwhelmed."

With the Lupron in his system, thwarted, compulsive lust was replaced by storms and floods of regret. It was as though desire, so rarely satisfied, had stymied everything else. Now, Berlin said, "He is no longer sitting in prison masturbating to fantasies about strangling someone." The medication, in the psychiatrist's mind, allowed the self to emerge, permitting

Ross his own humanity. Sorrow drowned him. He couldn't bear what he had done, couldn't endure the thought of the mothers and fathers of the dead being put through more waiting, more testimony, more memory, so he had started the campaign to quicken his execution. With sex eliminated, Ross became who he truly was.

BERLIN seemed, at times, to see Ross's new resolve as proof that sex and the self existed in opposition. Erotic desire wasn't the essence of the self; eros wasn't even essential to the self; Freud was far in the past. In expunging the libido, Lupron had liberated Ross's very being, his soul, and granted him excruciating guilt and the expiation of choosing death. It was at once a medical and religious vision, and Berlin was both a medical and religious man. The paraphilias were diseases, almost surely rooted in biology. He felt that the treatment he often prescribed—Depo Lupron or another anti-androgen, Depo Provera—was horribly imprecise. "It's a club," he said. The anti-androgens bludgeoned the hormonal foundation of desire rather than addressing specific aberrance. But he believed that, for now, until the brain was better understood and more delicate drugs were found, there was frequently no other choice. And once the medication spread through the system, redemption came quickly. The sexual sadist could become— purely—the good Samaritan who helped to change flat tires, and Michael Ross could become a man seeking his own sacrifice, asking to die for what he'd done.

"I pray to a god I cannot see; I depend on a god who may not be," Berlin said, smiling a bit sheepishly. He attributed the line to a patient from long in the past; he could not remember who. But the words had always stayed with him, and had become a credo of his own. The moment of uneasiness, as he acknowledged his measure of belief, seemed to arise from a feeling of unbelonging, an awareness that both the strictly religious and the devoutly scientific would scorn his statement of faith, the religious because he was far too tentative and the scientific because he depended on anything at all that was beyond the reach of proof and disproof. "I want there to be a higher power. I don't see that as a threat or alternative to science. I'm not going to be able to find a god, but as a human being I yearn. I desperately would like to believe, but if I'm really honest with myself, I'm just hoping that he's there."

Berlin affirmed what he could, proved what he could. The most depraved people were moral beings. With the aid of medicine, God, through a patient like Michael Ross, nearly came into view. Berlin worked with a necrophiliac who had a job at a funeral parlor; he treated a gynecologist voyeur. He welcomed uncountable pedophiles and child molesters into his office, invited them to his group therapy sessions, offered them— calmly urged upon them—medication. These, the most reviled of sex offenders, were the majority of his patients. Testifying in the state legislature, he fought against a mandatory reporting law that would require psychiatric professionals to notify the police if patients who came for treatment voluntarily, with no record of sexual offenses, confided incidents of abuse. Berlin didn't want a law that would deter the undetected from approaching him for help. In this way, he guarded his role as confessor, his ability to redeem, his immersion in the chaos of eros.

From that chaos he needed refuge. A huge and majestic saltwater aquarium was mounted in his office, dominating the room, the brilliant colors of the fish overwhelming the deep red of the antique furniture. A sea apple, like a purple and yellow balloon with white tentacles sprouting from the top, migrated slowly, searching for invisible particles of food. A surgeonfish, its blue scales set off by streaks of ebony, glided above pink coral. A yellow tang darted around a flaming red angel. Cowfish, with their strange horns and broad gray bellies, hovered above a crab, a clam. "Even that clam has an existence there," Berlin said, at once marveling at the thought of a clam's reality and laughing at his own wonderment. "And that sea apple—he moves to the front of the tank, where he can get the best nutrition. I don't know what in nonhumans constitutes a feeling or thought, but it would be very presumptuous of us to believe we're the only living entities capable of having some sort of subjective existence. To watch something like that, that almost looks like a balloon, and to see that it makes purposeful movements and has a life, it makes you think, it makes you wonder, and I find it very relaxing and very fascinating."

He liked simply to sit and stare into the tank, and to imagine a world of subjective experience that included no torment. He was mesmerized, too, by the compatibility of the underwater beings, the coral and crabs, the lone clam and all the species of fish. "Everything in there is alive, there's nothing artificial, and there's a symbiotic way in which they all survive together."

Within each creature, and for all of them combined, he perceived a tranquility denied to humans. "These species," he added, "rarely mate in captivity."

WHEN Jacob arrived, Berlin gave him the "Multiphasic Sex Inventory" and the "Million Clinical Multiaxial Inventory," two long questionnaires designed to elicit a patient's sexual preferences and his disorders of mind or mood. There were three hundred items on the sexual test, each requiring an answer of true or false: "Occasionally I think of things too bad to talk to others about. . . . I have exposed myself one hundred times. . . . It does not interest me to learn that a woman may not be wearing panties. . . . It would peak my interest to learn that a child is curious about sex. . . . I would like to be tied up and made to have sex." And there were one hundred and seventy-five more on the multiaxial. With his labored reading, Jacob took several hours to get through. "I can remember one of the questions was about interest in animals," he recalled. "And I'm thinking, *What?* That's disgusting. That's ridiculous. And then I thought, I'm a hypocrite."

He felt a degree of comfort in Berlin's mansion, partly because the façade bore no name, nothing to broadcast the perversions that brought people here; partly because he was now, for the first time in his life, ensconced within a world constructed for deviants like himself; and partly because he admired and trusted Berlin, though as Jacob struggled through the questionnaires the two men had scarcely talked. Jacob had formed an opinion based on the only thing he'd ever read about foot fetishism, a short article he'd come across in *Psychology Today*. The writer quoted Berlin saying that without attention to the feet the fetishist "usually can't get aroused"—from these and a few other words, Jacob felt that the psychiatrist was able to stare into his soul. Soon he would think of Berlin "like a god." And soon he would renounce going to synagogue, because he felt so betrayed by a god who could make him so alien. Berlin became his deity, soothingly Jewish, with a torah scroll sitting atop one of the bookcases in his office. The psychiatrist seemed all-knowing. He seemed unconditional in his forgiveness and sympathy. His mansion felt like Toronto, a haven.

Berlin reviewed the tests and called Jacob into his office to talk. Jacob showed him the copy he'd kept of the article from *Psychology Today*: an offering. The snow boots and socks and first memories of desire at the age of seven, the phone surveys taken sometimes several times in a day, the electric effect of the feet on the dashboard, the terror of late spring, the unendurable mortification—Jacob gave his history.

"I think I can help you," Berlin said.

"You do?"

The doctor talked of a patient drawn to earlobes, assuring Jacob that he was not so strange. "I think I can help," he repeated.

"I don't," Jacob said.

"I can't cure you. I don't want you to have false expectations, because this will always be there. But I can help." Berlin explained the anti-androgens, their effect on the sex drive, on physical arousal, and, too, their side effects, the possibility of developing breasts, the chance that his bone structure would weaken and warp.

Jacob was too desperate to take pause. "You might be able to control the physical, but not the mental," he insisted, trying not to hope, straining to protect himself against disappointment. "You can't control my thoughts." And it was his thoughts, as much as anything, that he wanted to purge. He wanted to poison their source in what felt like the center of his hideous being.

"You're wrong," Berlin said.

"I hope I'm wrong."

"You are. There will be a difference mentally."

Jacob thought, You're full of crap. You don't know how strong this is. He said, "I'll do whatever you tell me to do. I'll pay you whatever it is. I just can't take this anymore, I just can't be this way anymore. Just tell me what to do."

"I've never met someone so agreeable." Berlin laughed gently.

"Usually I have to fight with people."

"You're not going to have to fight with me."

BERLIN hardly knew why he'd begun to steer, in college in the 1960s, from psychology to psychiatry—and toward a vision that focused on the biological, that saw nature as a more promising area than nurture in which to search for understanding of the sexual mind. He recalled learning, as an undergraduate, about a scientist who was altering drives like thirst by implanting electrodes in the brain, and he remembered studying the Heinrich Kluver and Paul Bucy experiment on the brains of monkeys: the surgical lesions inflicted on the monkeys' temporal lobes, followed by the eruption of crazed sexual activity, not only with other monkeys but with an array of inanimate objects. And injury to the same region in the human brain could lead to the same sort of indiscriminate and unrestrained desire.

But in Berlin's own telling, there was no moment, or series of moments, of decision or inspiration that had formed his vision. He didn't seem to think in such terms. It was as though his way of seeing had happened to him for reasons impossible to know—exactly as he thought about the erotic directions of his patients. All the talk and introspection in the world couldn't unbury the causes. When Jacob asked, during their first meeting, "Why am I like this?" Berlin answered, "It's the way you're wired." When Jacob asked, at every meeting afterward, "Why? Why? I want an answer why. I need an answer why," Berlin gave the same response, sometimes adding rhetorically, "Why are people gay?" When Jacob tried Berlin with a theory offered by his first therapist, that back in the second grade, frantic to avoid being called on because he couldn't read, he'd kept his eyes on the floor, and that somehow, in those highly charged moments of yearning for escape, he'd started to eroticize his classmates' feet, Berlin dismissed it.

And probably most in his field had grown doubtful of experiential explanations. But his sexologist colleague at Hopkins and at the mansion, Greg Lehne, told me that the link to Jacob's second-grade classroom made "perfect sense. People's sexual interests are very specific. Scientists now are inclined to look at genetic or prenatal issues, but why people become lovestruck at certain qualities, why we're taken with a body type, or a shape of mouth or what a person's nose looks like, or an aspect of warmth or a sadistic side—where do these interests come from? They must come through experience, through the senses."

Lehne, with graying hair combed tightly back from a padded face, talked about how the prevalence of certain fetishes shifted with changes in the prevailing culture. Rubber fetishes had faded after the era of rubber training pants; hair fetishes had become less common as mothers and older sisters no longer made a ritual of letting down their tresses and brushing a prescribed number of times. It was impossible to quantify such shifts precisely, impossible to cite numbers for particular paraphilias, he said, but the changes could be traced by studying pornography and the hungers it catered to.

Lehne didn't fully discount the genetic, the prenatal, but the physiology of the brain was, he suspected, profoundly affected by what the mind took in. He studied paraphilias as a way to peer in at the workings of all desire, and mostly he saw the directions of eros as learned, not inborn. "The lovemap cartographic system," he had written, borrowing language from the legendary Hopkins psychologist John Money, "may operate like a multi-sensory camera that episodically takes photos of the immediate environment and stores them as depictions of the sexual terrain."

A young married couple had led Berlin to his career in sex. When he'd been a general psychiatric resident-in-training at Hopkins in the mid-seventies, a husband and wife had walked onto his ward. The husband carried a wooden club, about a foot long, with a heavy chain attached to it. They told of a guillotine-like hole he'd cut in their bedroom door. No permanent injury had been inflicted yet, but his fantasies were brutal, and their fear, Berlin remembered, was that "this was about to get very out of hand. He was afraid he would kill his wife, and she was afraid it could happen. They were simple people. She wasn't even sure how many couples did or didn't do this kind of thing."

When he tried to discuss the case with his supervisors and fellow residents, Berlin ran into trouble. They seemed repelled by the subject, and Berlin was criticized merely for quoting the man's crude language from his case notes, for reciting the phrase "jerk off." Acutely he sensed the particular taint that attached itself, even amid a group of psychologists and psychiatrists, "to anyone who acknowledged something different about their sexual makeup." He sensed a visceral unease with sex in general.

And hearing Berlin relate this story reminded me of an interview I'd done with a couples' counselor in Manhattan. She told me that she and a group of colleagues spoke often about the fact that not only in individual but in marital counseling sex is frequently the last thing the therapist asks about—and that the subject may never be raised at all.

Berlin still kept the club the husband had turned over. It lay in a hulking antique safe in the basement of his mansion. He'd treated the man with an anti-androgen, and, he said, the patient reported that his sadistic fantasies had faded away but that he could still become erect and function sexually. It was a long time ago, and it was impossible to know to what extent this had been true. That anti-androgens could attack the sex drive in such a way as to neutralize a paraphilia while leaving some degree of conventional desire and potency intact was unusual but known to happen. Nothing about the brain's and body's system of arousal was understood well enough, then or now, to predict when it would. No one could explain it. Understanding of the forces of eros was as crude as the original comprehension of testosterone itself, a hundred and fifty years ago, when a German zoologist had snipped off the testes of young roosters and watched their bright red combs atrophy along with their interest in nearby hens. If he took the severed balls and implanted them in a rooster's belly, all returned to normal, suggesting that the testes secreted a substance crucial to sexuality—a hormone that was discovered ninety years later by a Dutch scientist, who used almost a ton of bulls' testicles in isolating less than a third of a gram of testosterone.

After two or three years, the couple with the club drifted out of touch; Berlin never heard from them again. He had only the weapon as a memento of the case that had stirred his fascination and started him on his career. At Hopkins, John Money became an early mentor. A decade earlier, Money had taken on the case of a baby boy whose penis had been seared off in a botched circumcision. The parents worried that he would never be able to live as a man, and Money, a pioneer in his work with hermaphrodites and a believer that gender and sexual orientation are determined through social learning in early childhood, persuaded the parents to raise the boy, Bruce, as a girl, Brenda. Bruce's testicles were clipped, and a rudimentary vagina was constructed. Brenda took estrogen to help her grow breasts. Following his patient, Money wrote about her thriving as a girl, and the case was celebrated in *Time* magazine and in the *New York Times*.

He wrote, too, about paraphilias, cataloging and often coining the names of all the types, from acrotomophilia, "a paraphilia of the stigmatic/eligibilic type in which sexuoerotic arousal and facilitation or attainment of orgasm are responsive to and dependent upon a partner who is an amputee," to zoophilia, the desire for an animal. The paraphilias were, in Money's view, imprinted in childhood; they were the product of learning more than biology, nurture more than nature. Considering why sexual deviations are, so far as scientists know, mostly limited to the human species, he pointed to the sophistication of the human brain. Erotic "diversity," he explained, "may be an inevitable evolutionary trade-off—the price paid for the freeing of the primate brain to develop its uniquely human genesis of syntactical speech and creative intelligence."

Money's thinking was defiantly humane. He spoke about men like Jacob, and about sexual sadists and necrophiliacs and pedophiles, as people living not merely with deviant lust but with "disorders of love." He was willing to apply to paraphiliacs the typical connections between initial desire, falling in love, and long-term "pairbonding." He might have argued that, condemned by his condition, a man like Michael Ross was searching not only for sex but for love, in his murderous way. He talked about the tenderness and love often felt by pedophiles for their victims; he insisted that these emotions had validity and could be returned. "If I were to see the case of a boy aged ten or eleven who's intensely erotically attracted toward a man in his twenties or thirties, if the relationship is totally mutual, and the bonding is genuinely totally mutual, then I would not call it pathological in any way."

Berlin was taken with the complexity and bravery of his mentor's ideas, but he was more tempered in his thinking, and he never shared Money's faith in the importance of nurture over nature. He felt, now, that time had proved him right. Brenda, with her surgically built semblance of a vagina, and with her drug-induced breasts, had, despite Money's published reports, never taken on a girl's psyche, though she'd been brought up as a girl by her parents and never told about the circumciser's accident and psychologist's experiment that had decided her gender. She had refused to have further surgery to construct more complete genitalia. She felt alien and violent and distraught, and at last, when she was fourteen, her father confessed all that had been done. Soon Brenda set out to become a man, to become what biology had made her. She underwent a double mastectomy. She had a penis and testicles created from grafts and plastic. She injected testosterone to give herself a man's muscles. She named herself David. And eventually David killed himself.

Berlin talked about this failure, and another—with pedophiles. "Money was the first person to use medicines to lower testosterone. His theory back then, and I hope I'm doing justice to it, was that you give people a vacation from their sexuality and that gives psychotherapy time to work. Myself and some other researchers, with his permission, we took a look at the outcomes. And what we found was that as long as the people were still taking the medicine they were not reoffending, but a very high percentage who had the psychotherapy—once they stopped the medicine they did reoffend. We now don't look at the medication as a treatment while you're waiting for psychotherapy to work; it's more like insulin for diabetes. This is what you need over the long haul to keep you in control of yourself."

Thinking about the sources of particular desires—Michael Ross's for the sadistic; Jacob's for feet; the most prosaic erotic preferences of the most prosaic heterosexual—Berlin acknowledged the potential role of childhood experience but couldn't much credit it. The connections seemed loose and unlikely ever to be conclusively demonstrated. He believed that the sources would eventually be found, primarily, in the realm of biology, that they would prove to be "programmed in," as technology advanced to better illuminate the brain. He lamented the loss of free will that his prophesy seemed to imply, worried that such biological determinism supplanted the idea of mind as opposed to brain, feared an Orwellian world where neurological understanding would be precise enough so that the sexual regions of the brain could be manipulated to eliminate variations of desire or so that sexual anomalies could be detected in the womb and fetuses could be aborted accordingly—but the truth of biology's inborn power seemed inescapable.

To Berlin, the only solution with someone like Jacob was to fight biology on its own terms, no matter how crude the weapon—to prescribe an anti-androgen and hope that, with lust obliterated, Jacob would find within himself at least a faint version of conventional longings. This had happened not only with the sadist who'd handed Berlin his club but, more recently, with another patient. Berlin's gynecologist voyeur, who'd lost his practice and barely avoided prosecution before coming to Berlin for help, told me that on Lupron sheer lust was completely killed but that other yearnings—for pleasing a partner, for conforming to the society's notion that a married couple should be having sex—continued to motivate. "The skin on skin," he added. "The feelings of being close to someone. And the orgasm still feels good. Though you're not fired up by the primitive side of your brain. So sex can seem a very messy thing, like more trouble than it's worth, like why bother." He mentioned that he used Viagra, which Berlin prescribed for some of his patients on anti-androgens, patients who'd gotten control of relatively harmless paraphilias, so that, devoid of the urgency of lust, they might be able to become erect and carry out their more tender longings. He mentioned, too, that his penis had shrunken slightly since he'd started taking Lupron. Then he laughed: "I wonder what would happen if all men went on it for six months. Think about the advertising industry. All those commercials aimed at the primitive sexual urge. They'd have to find a new way to sell SUVs and beer."

Berlin, thinking about the experience of men like the gynecologist, told me: "I guess the distinction I'd make would be between eating to satisfy an intense hunger versus eating to enjoy the taste of food. These guys, on the Lupron, are not responding to a hunger to have sex, but sex can still feel good; they can still enjoy that taste."

He couldn't know whether Jacob, on Lupron, would feel any wish at all for sex, any inclination to eat for taste, with hunger gone. But he felt compelled to prescribe the drug. He felt certain that he should wipe out the hunger, though Jacob had harmed no one.

ONE evening, several years after meeting Berlin and starting Lupron, Jacob led a support group for the bipolar and the depressed. He'd founded the group himself, with the help of his city's mental health association, and he'd since become president of the association's board. Tonight, with the March snowbanks high, he laid out pizzas and cookies and pamphlets on a Formica table. He always left home early for the twice-monthly group meetings, allowing enough time to buy food and get everything neatly set up before the members arrived. The thirty or so pamphlets, along with booklets and flyers, explained an array of emotional disorders and their possible remedies, from aromatherapy to treatment with electroshock. In the few years since he'd started the group, Jacob had never missed a meeting. In the worst blizzards, he'd dug out his car and made it to the office building that had donated a basement conference room to his cause. Shoveling out his driveway, he was pushed on by the worry that a lone member would be waiting in the snowy parking lot, despondent, abandoned.

Four long beige tables were arranged in a square, and tonight all of the twenty-five chairs were taken. "We have a fairly large group this evening," Jacob said, beginning efficiently within a few minutes of the scheduled time, "so we're going to have to stay on track." The members introduced themselves, going around the square, and so did two visitors, psychology majors from a nearby college. Then a woman spoke of skipping her pills and becoming delusional and seeing knives that tried to coax her to cut herself to shreds. "I wasn't like this four years ago till I had the car accident," she said. "People at work say, 'Can't you just snap out of it?'"

"People just can't understand it," Jacob affirmed quietly, soothingly.

Another woman wondered aloud about electroshock, first for the woman seeing knives, then for herself. Jacob confided to everyone that he'd had the therapy. "It's not what it was. It's not the barbaric treatment you see in *One Flew Over the Cuckoo's Nest* or *A Beautiful Mind*."

Verging on catatonic, with matted blond hair, a college-age

girl complained about the group sessions her therapist had told her to attend at a state facility "with people less fortunate than me." It was clear that she couldn't bear to sit with patients she saw as more lost than herself. "I just want to skip past this phase and be normal," she said, her voice a hollow monotone. "Do I need to go?"

"Yes," Jacob answered. "Yes, yes you do. It's important to get out of the house. It's important not to isolate." He took off his watch and set it in front of him, mindful of the time so that everyone who wished would have the chance to speak.

"Today is my birthday," a man who was attending for the first time shared. "And this group is my treat to myself. I am in some pain, I am in some pain."

"Happy birthday," Jacob said softly, when the man had finished explaining the harrowing emotional journey that had led him here.

"Happy birthday," the group echoed, welcoming him.

A bipolar man said that his medication was running low, that there were problems with his insurance. A woman offered some of her pills. "No," Jacob cautioned. "See me after. I'll point you in the right direction. We can get that problem addressed."

Someone asked about the Vagus Nerve Stimulator, and Jacob explained how it worked. The battery-powered generator was implanted in the chest; electrodes were threaded to the neck, to where the vagus nerve ran up into the brain stem; the pulsations of current seemed to temper depression.

"I've joined a writing group," a young woman announced. "I'm working on three novels, and I've got some short stories." She allowed that she didn't fully trust her current optimism, that she wondered if she was entering a manic phase.

"Manic!" people called out, laughing knowingly. "Manic!"

"The first time I became manic," a partially toothless black woman joined in, "this was a good ways back, I was hitchhiking down the main drag in Houston dressed—how do you call it?—voluptuous, on my way to a lip-synching contest, thinking that's how I can make some money. And the police picked me up for a hooker. So there I was in the clink, saying, 'I'm not a hooker, I'm a lip-syncher.'"

"Well, there's *your* novel," a man said.

Everyone howled.

"It's just nice to be around people who get it," a woman said.

"Happy birthday," the newcomer mouthed, wishing it to himself, welcoming himself.

JACOB had created this twice-monthly world, and he conducted it as though his own agony was in the past. No one in the group knew that he was so tortured by his sexuality that he chose to eliminate it. No one knew that the electroshock he'd described, which he'd had both before and since Berlin, was an attempt to get free of a keen and relentless depression with sex enmeshed at its source.

Berlin had been right in at least one way. Lupron's attack on testosterone, on this single hormone, had been an attack on his thoughts. It wasn't only that physical arousal seemed to fade from possibility. The fantasies evanesced as well, along with the constant awareness of feet, the constant susceptibility to desire. A profound shift in consciousness occurred, as though the mind had emptied itself of eros.

Yet the emptying wasn't quite complete. Eros lingered and lurked, allowing him hours of numb tranquility and then edging forward to seize him with a yearning that was no less painful for being slightly abstract. A commercial on TV contained a scene of barefoot teenagers. A young saleswoman asked to measure his son's feet when Jacob took him to buy ski boots. At such moments his longing was perhaps even greater than it had once been, because the possibility of release was remote. He wasn't going to masturbate at the first opportunity, as he would have in the past. He wasn't going to explode without touch. He no longer grew hard easily, and he wouldn't permit himself to work himself up. He forbade himself to masturbate. Seeing the barefoot teenagers on TV, he slammed his fist down onto his coffee table.

Sex with his wife was gone entirely. He didn't know what she understood about the desire he drugged into submission. He'd always evaded candor, and Berlin, at their first long meeting, had advised that he keep things vague. She seemed to collude in his omissions.

He had tried Viagra in high doses. It didn't help. Jacob thought that if he focused on his wife's feet, if he gazed at them and caressed and clutched them, he would generate enough craving to overcome the Lupron and grow hard, especially if he added Viagra. But he wanted nothing to do with these grotesque pleasures, and the Lupron diminished his drive sufficiently so that he could succeed in self-denial. He didn't gaze, didn't caress. Her feet remained under the covers when they attempted to make love. He stayed soft. They stopped trying.

It was Greg Lehne and another of Berlin's colleagues, Kate Thomas, who told me that people like Jacob are not merely cursed, that they possess a special capacity for ecstasy. "There's no comparison between what they experience and normal sexuality," Lehne said. "It's a hyper-positive sexual experience." And Thomas added, "I don't think we, in our sex lives, have a hint of what they feel." One explanation, in Jacob's case,

was that in his second-grade classroom his anxiety about being called on reached the level of full-blown panic attacks—as
he'd aimed his eyes downward, his fear was reconfigured as
sexual arousal that was equally extreme. But Lehne stressed
that this was only theory; the reasons, in all cases, remained
mysterious.

With a paraphilia that was harmless, Lehne and Thomas
felt that their primary role was to listen; their hope for the
patient was self-acceptance. Cure—in the form of the trans-
formation of desire—might never be possible, but a measure
of peace could be reached. To treat someone like Jacob meant
trying to lift the shame and to incorporate the focus of desire
into the marriage.

Why couldn't his wife's feet be shown and gazed upon,
flaunted and craved, offered and touched? Why couldn't these
gestures and responses sometimes be part of foreplay and other
times lead to the pairing of her feet and to his penetrating
between them? Weren't analogous things done with breasts
and buttocks? Weren't they put on display in all manner of
clothes and swimsuits and lingerie, to be stared at and reached
for? Why couldn't feet be objectified and included in the erotic
life—and in the love live—of a couple, just as the common
secondary sexual characteristics were incorporated between
so many men and women?

"'I've got three shit dates lined up in one weekend.'" Winston
Wilde, a psychologist in Los Angeles, told me that a patient, a
coprophiliac, had just spoken these words to him. Wilde didn't
disparage his patient's wish to be smeared with or eat a partner's feces. He quoted the man in a celebratory, even exultant
tone, as an emblem of therapeutic success. "A big aspect of sex
therapy is permission-giving," he said. "It's important to give
an education. Sometimes people's whole lives can change if

you direct them to an Internet site. I always like to normalize their situation."

Berlin didn't talk much in terms of "permission-giving." It was hard to imagine him advertising a patient's "shit dates" as evidence of successful therapy. He did hope that one day he would be able to help Jacob and his wife toward erotic intimacy, but the eros he envisioned seemed to have nothing to do with feet. For all the compassion in his thinking, Berlin seemed no more willing to accept Jacob's desire than Jacob was himself. When I asked him, at one point, about the possibility of encouraging Jacob and his wife to include her feet as a spark to intimacy, he didn't really answer the question, and when I pressed, he said, "I think Jacob is somewhat content not having sex at all and doesn't necessarily feel deprived."

I'd heard nothing like this from Jacob. I'd heard him describe slamming his fist onto his coffee table. I'd heard him tell about trying to go off Lupron against Berlin's advice. He'd stopped the medication for a short period, but self-revulsion over his desire had chased him back onto the drug. Knowing about this attempt, Berlin nevertheless suggested that Jacob didn't mind living without sex. It sometimes seemed he was driven, consciously or not, to medicate aberrant lust out of Jacob's life.

Then Jacob decided to try once more to go without the injections. He pushed the experiment to a year, but still couldn't bring himself to open up to his wife about his longing. "Because it's not normal! Because it's not right! Because I love her!" he answered when I asked, again, why. He would not taint her with his perversity, include her in his monstrosity; instead, he mortified himself all the more with a series of prostitutes until he crawled back to Berlin and the Lupron.

After this second attempt, Berlin spoke to me in more ambivalent terms about Jacob's treatment. "Because his situation is less dangerous than others', because it poses little threat, it's harder to make a decision about what should be done, about whether to medicate or not." But in the end, Berlin believed it was necessary, that it was the less painful option for his patient. He spoke about "freeing up the mind from sex. When we're young, eliminating sex may be inconceivable, but when we're older we may find that it's more peaceful, that companionship is more fulfilling. If we're hungry we want to eat, but if we're not we may not miss it."

Berlin talked as well about anti-androgens as an antidote, for patients like Jacob, to the tendency to "objectify women"—talk that sounded enlightened. But did Jacob objectify any more than any man? Or did a difference like his simply spotlight what was universal? To be drawn to a woman's feet, to isolate such an odd body part, was, it could seem, to dissect her, to give physical attraction a brutal primacy. To be lured by breasts or legs or buttocks was to have base desire softened by convention, blurred by normality—the body was left intact, along with the possibility of loving a woman's soul. The distinction was arbitrary. Jacob's desire put all desire under a glaring light, and the view, I sensed, made Berlin uncomfortable.

He had fought through all kinds of discomfort in his career. His compassion for sex offenders had brought vilification. His children had been teased by classmates because their father stood up for serial killers. But it was as though the stark physicality of desire, the animal aspect of it, was too much to face. He needed sex to be soulful, "human." Jacob's eros seemed to frighten him. Jacob was, in Berlin's eyes, thoroughly human. His lust was not.

• • •

"YOU'RE making me cry," Jacob said one afternoon. We sat in a restaurant in one of the other snowy cities along his salesman's route. The decor had a pioneer theme. Wagon wheels and paintings of buffaloes hung on walls made of knotted wooden planks. The waitresses wore gingham, and the shelves and buckets in the gift shop were filled with statuettes of cowboys and Native American chiefs. It was lunchtime, and the place was packed with men and women in crisp, informal work clothes: khakis, sensible skirts, sports jackets, high-collared blouses. Nothing in the way they looked suggested that their lives bore much similarity to Jacob's. And maybe very few of them were holding secretly anything like his agony. Yet Jacob dressed like them, worked in business like many of them, lived in a comfortable, modest home like many of them, and it was easy to think that many of them were consumed by invisible battles with their erotic selves, their central selves. The husband whose longing for other women had reached the point of daily pain; the wife whose yearning for someone or something else was just as excruciating; the middle-aged man who had never told anyone that he was gay and felt that it was far too late to reveal himself now; the young woman who craved violence in the faultlessly tender arms of her fiancé—they all ate their french fries amid the wagon wheels.

"You're making me cry," Jacob said, because I had asked him to imagine a world where almost all men—ninety-four percent was the number I picked out of the air—saw feet as the locus of desire. He removed his glasses, pinching the corners of his eyes and the bridge of his nose to stanch the welling tears. "How about those Yankees?" he joked to stop himself from breaking down. He waited to gain control before he spoke again.

In Toronto, he told me, he'd seen *The Phantom of the Opera* for the first of seven times. It was another reason the city was the place of his dreams. "Colm Wilkinson's singing," he said, recalling the actor who played the Phantom, "was the most beautiful thing I've ever heard in my life. I was shaking during some of those scenes." Jacob recounted the story of the hideously disfigured man who lives beneath the opera house in subterranean secrecy, thwarted in love. He quoted the Phantom's wail, "I've been denied the pleasures of life." He described waiting outside the theater's back door after the performance, the temperature below zero, to have Wilkinson autograph a poster. "I bought the tape and listened to it three thousand times," he said. Then, for a while, he was silent.

"I can't imagine being in the ninety-four percent. It would be like I was able to climb up and live in the world."

PART II

THE BEACON

DURING THE ABU GHRAIB PRISON SCANDAL, THE Baroness received a flood of phone calls. The photographs that ran in the newspapers and on television, the images and descriptions of torture, especially the picture of an Iraqi standing on a box with a hood over his head and electrical cables running to his hands, stirred a surge of requests. Could she do that for the caller, inflict that kind of fear followed by jolts of electricity?

She was a clothing designer. Her sheath-like outfits had been featured in full-page liquor ads on the backs of magazines. Janet Jackson, newly thin, had posed in her clothes. So had Kim Basinger. Music video dancers snaked and twisted in her outfits. A kimono she'd embroidered long ago, when she'd worked with a different aesthetic, hung in the Smithsonian Museum. Her boutique was a narrow storefront in Manhattan's East Village, and in the basement, with its brick walls painted mint green and its tightly wedged worktables, she and her submissives constructed the garments.

Her clothing lines were all latex. She liked to show her submissives how to create a seam, setting one piece of material upon another, with adhesive between, and running a finger precisely, sensually, along the overlap. "Latex is a physical thing," she said. "When I teach someone how to make a garment I teach them about touch. I teach them how to take their finger and *lay* down the seam. Don't press too hard and don't press too soft. Just feel it."

Her basement was a place of pleasure, of lashing, burning, beating, cutting, gagging, branding. "My lips swell," she described what happened when she gave pain. "My heart beats quickly, I'm sure my pupils dilate. I feel massive." She stood at a worktable as she spoke, her eyes closed. Her hair was a stiffly teased conflagration of red and blond hues, like a tumbleweed bursting perpetually into flame. "I stay away from small equipment. I don't allow myself a scalpel. With a scalpel I might just pop it straight through. Skin, muscle, organs. I feel like God. There is a stillness when I'm about to use the bullwhip, or my wand if I'm to set someone on fire. Have you ever watched an animal that is scared, caught in headlights or conscious of your presence, and scared—it just stops. And you, watching, you can feel time stopping. Stopping. It's not just the animal, it's time; the animal sucks time out of the air. And you stand there listening to something that isn't there."

She wore a ruby red latex dress, cut low and pushing high at the bust, the lacing in back drawn tight. A metal leaf arrangement, fashioned from part of a candleholder, protruded from her hair. She wore emerald-green eye shadow, and as her eyes remained shut while she described her experience, her eyelids—parched and pebbled with middle age—trembled.

The clothes she sold tended to be minimalist in their lines, but some were as flamboyant as she herself never failed to be.

She felt she belonged to an era more than half a century past; she drew inspiration from the thirties and forties. She had just begun work on a floor-length gown whose wide shawl collar and ruffled sleeves would be thick with lace—except that she would use only latex. And this posed a technical problem. Latex is perfectly suited to cling, to encase, to lie thin and flat. It doesn't serve well in creating volume, let alone in replicating blooms and clouds of lace, which was the effect the Baroness had in mind.

She stared at the sketch she had drawn, in which the woman's face was partly obscured by a bit of veiling that descended from her hat—the hat and veiling, too, would be latex. She contemplated her dilemma. How to make lace from latex? It was the kind of question she liked to consider; for all her sense of fashion, she proclaimed herself a "geek." She would stare and experiment, toss away and sketch and contemplate again. The insoluble generally got solved. She saw in her own way. "Arrange these," she said to me, upstairs in her boutique. She pointed to a latex flower in silver and amethyst, a postcard, a figurine, a pliable bit of orange cable, and a few other small objects that happened to lie on the glass counter. I set about making formations, this next to that: simple patterns in two dimensions. The possibilities seemed limited. Then she took over. She bent objects around each other, entwined them, melded them, thus making new things. She saw that, with each other, the objects could be transformed.

She was that way with people. She was an evangelical sadist, offering revelation and aiming to shape a new world. Jacob couldn't find a place for himself within the world that existed. The Baroness intended to create a world that was her place. "To have someone new is marvelous," she said in her faint British accent. Her speech combined the clipped and the dramatic, the precise and the ethereal. "To watch the body go from stiffness, from fear, to watch it giving way and leaning into the whip. Once we reach that point I could be in a room of two hundred people, I'm not aware of their presence. I go basically deaf. Wine. The smell of a certain wine: your grandmother's cheek and blackberries. It rushes over you. It is as delicate as that, but so strong that nothing else can intrude."

She was happily married, a conventional union of twenty years. She had been collecting disciples for a decade. "I tell them I provide a safe place to do dangerous things. But that is a lie."

THE doorbell rang, and the Baroness buzzed the customer in. He had a rim of gray hair and a British accent far stronger than hers. He asked to try on a black bodysuit. She instructed him in how to apply a body lubricant called Eros, which would allow him to slide the latex over his skin. "Okay," he said.

"It's not 'okay,'" she corrected in a voice at once understanding and stern. "It's 'Yes, Baroness.'"

"Yes, Baroness." He went behind the ice-blue satin curtain into the dressing room, its walls draped in satin of the same color. His sharp intakes of breath were audible throughout the boutique as he put on the lubricant and worked himself into the suit.

"I think I'm a submissive," he said through the curtain.

She let some moments pass. "You think or you know?"

He emerged, and she started to fit him, tugging and smoothing the material. He acknowledged that he knew.

"Are you service-oriented?" she asked.

In this way, or by referral or chance, she was gathering her flock. Some became slaves, others only followers. There was the Girl, known solely by this generic name in the basement workshop. A secretary in her early twenties, tall and chunky, with long brown hair parted in the middle, she had stepped into the boutique to shop several weeks earlier and been drawn to the Baroness right away. She was already owned by a man she'd met online, through Craigslist. But the man, it turned out, was willing to share her with a master whose reputation was national.

The Baroness had requested that formal papers be written up to delineate the terms of their co-ownership, and they met for dinner to discuss the details. The man's chief request was that he be invited to watch any bodily punishment. The Baroness was known for severity. But she had been holding back with the Girl: rigging her face with horse blinkers and a ball gag, binding her limbs, instructing two assistants to cane her. As she was caned, the Girl screamed in a choked-off, high-pitched way from behind the gag, which propped open her jaw at an impossible angle. Her eyes lost focus. The Baroness didn't take direct part in the beating, because the Girl was about to serve at her annual Christmas party, and the Baroness, who tended toward the extreme, didn't want her marked.

There was Frank, a window-washer, his face rugged below short brown bangs, handsome in the manner of a cigarette ad. He wore a black T-shirt, a creased and faded leather jacket. It was easy to place him in a common pornographic scene: washing a large bedroom window, then beckoned inside by the woman sprawled on the bed. When he arrived each afternoon at the boutique, he presented himself to the Baroness, as he'd been trained, just inside the front door: on his knees, arms tight to his sides and wrists bent back so that his palms and straightened fingers were parallel to the floor. His hands looked like paralyzed flippers. She would direct him to hold this posture for several minutes, correcting him if his wrists started to droop.

At last allowed to stand, Frank started to polish the front door's metal frame, a daily task, the weather quickly replacing any blemishes he managed to burnish away. As he polished, the mailman came. He and Frank said hello, exchanged pleasantries, a pair of simple working men.

"Have you rented *Remains of the Day*?" the Baroness asked Frank one afternoon. He'd just knelt before her, hands in position, to ask what his next task should be, after an hour at the door frame.

"No, Baroness. Forgive me, Baroness."

"You didn't expect me to ask?" Two weeks ago, she had instructed him to watch the story of the faultless, self-effacing butler.

"It's a hard movie to find, Baroness," he pleaded.

As he knelt, knees slightly splayed, she kicked him with terrific force in the testicles, connecting with the tip of her red boot. He shuddered and bent but made no sound. Next, he vacuumed the boutique. In the back pocket of his jeans he kept a small spiral notebook, as required, in order to take notes. "Please serve obey" were the words printed on one page. Another unpunctuated page read: "Always wear black when serving The Baroness never interrupt The Baroness always clean the front of the shop sweep wipe down never talk to The Baroness eye to eye." She commanded that her "the" be capitalized. For their own names her submissives adopted the lowercase. On a third page: "When trying to get The Baroness's attention always be in position to accept any discipline The Baroness feels I deserve."

After vacuuming, he returned to his knees to pour her a glass of champagne in the basement. Another trainee was

bathing her feet in a little plastic tub before giving her a pedi-
cure. The Baroness thought the pedicurist was more promising
than Frank; she considered the pedicurist a slave-in-training
while she doubted that Frank would ever rise above the level of
servant. "The cerulean blue," she said, choosing a color for her
toenails. A pretty young apprentice named Lara, whose father
was an executive at a billion-dollar food company, and whom
the Baroness often led around the city on a leash, leaned over
a worktable, making a pillbox hat. There was a technical problem. The latex wasn't providing enough structure. She brought
the hat to the Baroness, and they stared together at the inter-
nal band, talking over the design—colleagues.

The Baroness directed Frank to move a cabinet from a
corner of the workshop, her tone straightforward, not harsh.
She said that the pedicurist should join him. Within their two-
man team, Frank took easy charge. "You just lift," he said in a
street-corner accent, nonchalant, confident. "One, two, three."
Deeper into his notebook, he'd written: "Reasons why I want
to serve The Baroness. To fix her seamed stocking while she
cracks her bullwhip. To make things easier for The Baroness
so she can devote more time to her fashion business and make
more money and be happier, because she took her valuable time
to train me to be the best slave she can ever have. To learn how
to take The Baroness 16 bullwhips and never complain or cry."

ON a worktable one evening, a man lay on his back in a red
latex bodysuit and a black hood whose only openings were a
pair of grommets at the nostrils. Blue ropes, run through large
metal eyes at the rim of the table, held him down while a small
black machine sent an electrical charge to a conductive ring
around the shaft of his penis. The Baroness set the machine

to respond to voices, told the man to tell me about himself, and closed the French doors on that section of the basement. Whenever the man or I spoke, the current surged, and when he groaned or screamed in pain, the voltage went even higher. She had made me complicit in his torture.

He had retired from Wall Street a few years ago, in his mid-forties. He'd wanted to spend more time with his children, who were in their teens, and now he helped them with their homework and watched Fred Astaire movies with his daughter. His wife, a homemaker who had once had a practice as a psychologist, inflicted pain in their bedroom, but not with the same spirit as the Baroness. His feet quivered, then flapped as the voltage soared.

"It's about surrendering your ego," he said, sounding as though he must be gritting his teeth behind the hood. "The first time, after forty-five minutes, I was in another world. It was like onion skins were being peeled off my psyche." He talked about studying Plato, Nietzsche, and Kierkegaard in his retirement. His feet shook so hard it seemed his Achilles tendons might rupture. The Baroness would hold him captive this way for at least twenty-four hours, maybe thirty-six. When the boutique and the workshop closed, she would switch the electrical machine from voice-activated to random, and leave him bound and alone for the night. I wondered about going to the bathroom.

"You either don't or you make a mess or she applies a Texas catheter. This would be up to the Baroness to decide."

She told one of her acolytes to start shutting things down. It was around nine o'clock. No one would return until noon. I asked about his childhood.

"I was never raped by homosexual dwarves," he mocked my question. "Is this a weird way to deal with life? Consider the man who bought Mark McGwire's seventieth home-run ball for three million dollars. Who's weirder?"

GENEVIEVE she'd met at a fashion show. One of the Baroness's models hadn't shown up, and Genevieve had taken her place at the last minute. The Baroness sensed something about her, and soon they were out on a date at a mainstream movie theater, where the Baroness taped Genevieve's wrists to the armrests, taped her feet together, taped her mouth. It was the beginning of one of the great loves of her life, coexisting with her love for her husband. Genevieve couldn't serve the Baroness in her boutique or in her workshop, not productively, because they could never resist the temptation to "play." The transcendence that came with inflicting pain depended on a depth of connection—physical, emotional, spiritual—with the one she was hurting. The Baroness had plenty of quick encounters that gave shallow pleasure, and she had an array of regular submissives who might give her slightly more. She and Genevieve had been created for each other; there was a feeling of destiny between them; and now, several years after Genevieve had left New York and gone home to Canada to resume college, the longing that came with remembering left an emptiness in every artery, every vein. Thinking back, the Baroness shut her eyes against the loss, as though her eyelids could keep the void at bay. She could scarcely say what had lain beneath the attachment, only that it had been grounded in something more than the ferocity of their play. Once, as the Baroness lashed Genevieve's vulva, the end of her whip caught on the hoop ring Genevieve wore in her clitoris and ripped the hoop out through the glistening tissue.

• • •

THERE were psychologists who wouldn't have thought the Wall Street retiree or Genevieve or the Baroness herself were pathologically weird at all—or, if they did catch themselves thinking it, would swiftly have cautioned themselves against subjective judgment. "Perversion," Muriel Dimen, a prominent New York psychoanalyst, joked as we sat in her Greenwich Village office, "can be defined as the sex that you like and I don't." And Mark Blechner, editor of the journal *Contemporary Psychoanalysis*, said, "Remember that a century ago psychoanalysts were talking about fellatio and cunnilingus as perversions. As long as what she does is consensual," he went on, after I'd described the Baroness's life, "I don't think it's anyone's role to judge."

Dimen, whose dark gray ringlets of hair brightened suddenly to a dramatic white rim around her face, mentioned that perversion, in one current psychiatric conception, is characterized by "relationships in which relatedness disappears," but added that sadists and masochists may feel a resonant union. Erotic excitement, she had written, can send "you into bodily and sensory realms of abjection foreclosed long ago in the necessities of maturation." She used "abjection" in a psychoanalytic sense, to mean an infantile state before the boundaries of identity are formed—and to listen to the Wall Street retiree talk about surrendering and having onion skins stripped from his psyche, or to listen to the Baroness recall the violent and blissful merging of selves that had taken ungovernable hold whenever she and Genevieve were in the same room, was to hear a hint of the profound, the unbounded.

Dimen was reluctant to speak about causes of sadism or masochism; she worried about implying that such desires were disorders. But other psychoanalysts were less hesitant to see pathology. Doris Silverman, her hair dyed a soft, calming wheat-like shade, suggested that some lack of parental bond, some wounding absence or brutality, probably lay behind the sexual drives of people like the Baroness and those who submitted to her. Even Blechner, who refused to judge, suspected that the Baroness was responding to some long-repressed cruelty in her childhood. Then again, he warned that such psychoanalytic explanations had proved misguided in the past, that schizophrenia had once been attributed to cold and rejecting mothering.

EVAN worked with computers and was the president of his local Lions Club. Under his leadership, the club raised money to combat diabetes and childhood eye diseases. He served in the apartment the Baroness shared with her husband, cleaning and running errands and bringing her coffee in bed. He slept on her floor. A friend of his, who would soon become the first American reporter killed by insurgents in Iraq, had introduced him to the Baroness. She told me: "I love that people will come to me and say, 'You changed my life.' If you can leave a legacy of people better than they were before, you're blessed. I'm blessed in that way."

Other slaves she found by advertising in downtown newspapers. Applicants were instructed to arrive for an interview with a résumé detailing any previous service. Kneeling for her questions, one man explained that he had made, from scratch, the paper for the résumé he offered her.

Alex lived in a distant city. He phoned the Baroness at precise moments throughout the day—12:55, 3:37, 8:12— according to her commands and their synchronized watches. At each call, she told him what to do: bind himself more tightly, contort himself more unnaturally, burn himself. If he missed the time she assigned, her instructions might be more severe, or she might withhold punishment altogether, which was terrible in itself.

Sam was a contractor to the wealthy, the well known. He had waves of unkempt, shoulder-length brown hair and a way of wearing his T-shirts that communicated an indifferent self-assurance. As an offering, he did carpentry in the boutique, which had opened not long ago; he had made the elegantly curved counter, and he waited for the harm she might give. Susan, his wife, taught science in the New Jersey public high school from which she'd graduated twelve years earlier. She had jet-black hair, a delicate nose, full lips, a slender body; the Baroness used her for a model.

The couple had never lacked for heat between them. The first time they'd slept together, on a summer night, he'd gone to his freezer and taken out the tangerine sections he kept frozen there to run over a lover's nipples and thighs till they melted and were eaten. Later they'd seen the Baroness interviewed on HBO and ventured to her shop to buy each other latex outfits. A three-way flirtation had begun, and along the way the Baroness learned that Susan had endured a childhood illness that had left her back heavily scarred. Hearing about them, seeing them, the Baroness was enamored of those marks. "I'm somebody she looks up to, somebody she trusts," the Baroness said to me. "Everybody else tries to tell her, 'It's okay, they're not too bad.' I want to make her a dress to show off her back. I like the marks of life. Hers are massive. Marvelous, thick, like a ladder. You could climb down her back on those scars." And Susan told me that the Baroness was beginning to transform her.

Even those who hadn't entered the Baroness's world, even

near strangers, seemed to feel altered by her attention. A crippled teenage boy drove his motorized wheelchair along the blocks near her boutique. His neck sagged, his head keeled, his knees leaned together. His wrist was inverted over the chair's little black driving knob. But when he saw the Baroness stepping toward him in her sidewalk-length rubber coat, with her purple spiked heels, her fireball of hair, which sometimes contained a streak of white or magenta to complement the flames, her many silver rings, two or three to a finger, and her sleek iron cane, which she carried as an accessory and which looked like a gallant's sword, all obliterating her age, making the nascent pouches of her face irrelevant, making any measure of prettiness irrelevant, substituting flagrance for conventional standards so that, even in the East Village, where the outlandish was banal, every eye turned toward her—when he saw her approaching his face brightened and, though perhaps it wasn't possible, his neck seemed to straighten slightly, his head to lift.

"Hello, Baroness."

"Hello."

It was the same with the woman who walked with forearm crutches, the same with another woman, who seemed not quite homeless but plainly dislodged, as disheveled in her mind as in her hair and clothes.

"Hello, Baroness."

"Hello."

Sometimes, on the streets in the evening, she stopped to chat. Then the forearm crutches seemed momentarily unnecessary; the dishevelment disappeared, replaced by intriguing idiosyncrasy.

The effect might have been due to her flaunting her difference, to their recognizing a champion misfit. But she claimed another power. She said it was because she was willing to look at them. Most people averted their eyes from the crippled and avoided the lost. She, strutting loudly in her spiked heels along a line as straight as her iron cane, gazed not only into their eyes but at their bodies and into their minds. To do anything less, to pretend not to notice, was, she felt, to cause shame rather than diminish it. She was willing to see them, without fear, exactly as they were, and that freed them, for a few seconds, to be themselves.

ONE torrential Saturday afternoon the Baroness took me up-state for an overnight gathering hosted by her friend Master R. I picked her up outside her apartment building, and her husband, Mark, walked her out to the car. He had a sharp nose and a sharp chin, a ponytail and a goatee, and the grace-ful reserve of men with plenty of height. A photographer, he kept his distance from her world, except to take pictures at the monthly parties she threw. That was as close as he wanted to get. He preferred to take portraits of dogs, which he consid-ered his calling. He'd started a Web site, phodography.com, to advertise his vision: "Your dog is unique. (S)he is loyal. (S)he provides heart-healing humor and unconditional companion-ship. We understand completely." He and the Baroness had been married almost a decade before she'd discovered herself. He was still perplexed. Before we drove off he leaned down to her open window; they kissed warmly, devotedly. "Good-bye, handsome," she said.

On a hushed country road, Master R lived in a run-down bungalow he called La Domaine Esemar. There were deep puddles in the bald front yard and a feeling of manginess in the rooms within. He was a short version of Mark: a ponytail, piercing features. Wearing black velvet pants, he apologized to the Baroness, saying that because of the downpour the turn-out might be slim—his guests tended to drive long distances from other rural towns. Then he led us down to the basement and introduced us to those who were there: a cherubic Asian car salesman; the owner of a restaurant chain and his wife, a hospital administrator; a transsexual in a black slip of a dress, with lush lips and large teeth.

Aside from the exposed air ducts, the basement was the best-kept part of the house. All was clean and orderly. On blond shelves sat an endless variety of clips and clamps and stainless steel weights to be attached to testicles—all polished and gleaming and aligned in tidy rows. A black box, its bottom cut out, dangled from the ceiling so that a submissive could stand with her head inside. From facial piercings, her lips and tongue, ears and nose and eyebrows could be stretched and fastened to screw eyes that lined the inside of the box. To larger screw eyes on the outside, her wrists could be hooked, so that her hands would remain for hours and hours at the height of her ears. The box hung directly above a revolving platform on the floor. The submissive would be sent spinning with her head in darkness, her hands latched helplessly, and her face stretched to the point of tearing.

There was a red cross, a trellis of whips, a chandelier of chains from which to suspend subjects, a dentist's chair, a doc-tor's examining bed. Plastic sippy cups, the kind toddlers drink from, were lined on a shelf "in case a slave loses consciousness and needs water," Master R said.

The Asian Chevrolet salesman started to bind Lara, the Baroness's often-leashed apprentice, who had come along with us. Using heavy rope, he created a delicate corset, then cinched it tighter and tighter around her ribs like the stepmother suffocating Snow White. The artistry of Japanese bondage, he said, had begun centuries ago, when Samurai policemen devised elaborate ways of roping prisoners according to their social status. The restaurant owner and Master R listened while lashing the transsexual's back. Wispy streaks of new blood crossed lines of old scabs. She gave out deep groans of arousal, lips and teeth parted wide. Her head lolled forward and wagged. Her groans reached orgasmic levels. They lashed her thighs, which trembled, then pushed her down on all fours. Master R pinned her head to the concrete floor with his boot. She groaned from a yet more central place, utterly animalistic.

The Baroness was unmoved. "There isn't going to be any oneness for me tonight," she muttered; no one here would desire the extremity of pain she needed to give. Two years ago, in Master R's backyard, she had roasted a horse buyer named Elvis on a revolving spit.

Soon the hospital administrator, unclothed, had her ankles and wrists tied to a pair of freestanding poles, which were held upright, one by her husband and the other by the car salesman. They leaned the poles backward slightly; if they let go she would crash to the floor, her skull cracking against the cement. A woman who'd just arrived in a diaphanous skirt put her mouth to the administrator's crotch. The administrator floated on air and trust as the woman began to lick.

Released by Master R, the transsexual told me that as a man she'd been a neo-Nazi skinhead with a wife, a five-year-old daughter and a two-year-old son, and a job as a computer specialist at a law firm. Her kids still called her Dadda, though she had injected spectacular doses of estrogen into her body, dropped from two hundred and fifteen to one hundred pounds, and had only the shrunken vestige of male genitalia, which would soon be surgically removed. "They'll always call me Dadda or Dad," she said. She wore a slender silver ring on each hand, one for each child. "They'll never come off."

As a male she'd been walking alone on a beach one afternoon, flooded with anti-depressants but sobbing and saying aloud, "God help me." She'd known for years she simply wasn't meant to be what she was. "That guy died that afternoon. When I was a neo-Nazi, I didn't hate people, I hated myself." She paused, contemplative, tranquil after the violence that had just enveloped her. "The beating here pulls out my inner female; it goes so deep; I want to receive. It's like heroin. It takes me from a high head space, down through all the levels, down to someplace at my core. Everything gets brighter. Everything gets amplified. This is where I learn the whole. I stay with Master R for the weekends. Leaving is agony. The other world is agony. I have a hard time coming down. I'm jonesing. The law firm was good enough to keep me on after the sex change, but this is where I belong. It's two different worlds, this and the vanilla. This one is totally alive. That one is dead."

Master R handed me his unpublished autobiography, and I went upstairs where there was enough light to read. Much was about the obliteration of boundaries, the annihilation of identity, the finding of a new, undelineated being through the giving and receiving of pain: "I slipped the ropes around her waist, pulled them tight, took the working end and ran it between her legs. I could almost see her lips engorge as the rope cut deeply into her labia. I felt my own cock swell in communication with her lust. Slipping my hand down I felt the wetness. My own pussy sighed in joyous communication and her cock hardened in my hand. I felt my nipples turn to hard little berries as the cock in my hand became rigid." And as twine stitched through her labia was pulled taut: "I rubbed my wetness against him and moaned in return, as I stroked my cock and rubbed my clit. We were both lost in the intensity of our metamorphosis."

No one had an easy time leaving at the end of their stays, he claimed. He talked of a young corporate lawyer's adjustment each time he walked out the bungalow's peeling front door and drove back to his life in Manhattan. "How can you go out into the world afterward? People are trembling physically."

The Baroness was not trembling. But she recalled the day with Elvis. They'd agreed that she would roast him, and she'd called Master R for assistance. One of his slaves, a welder, built a massive spit: huge bases supporting a metal pole that was about ten feet long, a wheel at one end and spoke handles at the other. It joined a vegetable garden behind the bungalow. Maple and birch trees rose around it, leaves in brilliant color on that bright autumn afternoon. Slaves spread coals onto the bed. Elvis, naked except for a leather jock, was led from the house blindfolded, strapped to the pole, basted with honey and ginger. The coals glowed; the spit was a foot or so above them.

Skin turned red, on the verge of blistering. Elvis screamed while around him the guests, masters and submissives, entered into an orgy of pain inflicted and received. Under the Baroness's direction, slaves turned the spit slowly. The roasting went on for three and a half hours. When the pole was at last raised away from the heat and Elvis removed from it, he couldn't stand upright. His eyes were glazed. He collapsed and was carried to bed, guests forcing him to drink water and trying to keep him from going into shock.

"My thighs press together just to think of it," the Baroness said. She spoke about the different kinds of orgasms she experienced in vanilla sex with her husband, to whom she was faithful as far as vanilla sex went, and in the rest of her erotic life, which some might not have recognized as sex at all: it involved no intercourse, no touching of breasts or genitals. The orgasms in conventional sex were "spikier." The others were far longer, deeper, left her half-blind, mostly deaf, mute, slack-jawed.

IN the S-M world, Master R told me, orgasms without typical sexual touching weren't uncommon, especially for women. He mentioned training a slave to climax when he brushed the roof of her mouth with his finger. And I thought of the woman I'd met after a lecture the Baroness had given, the speech therapist for stroke victims, who reviled her own orgasmic sensitivity: if a sadistic lover whispered in her ear in the right way, she could come without any touch beyond the grazing of his breath. An Orthodox Jew whose grandparents had been slaughtered in the Holocaust, she felt tormented by her own craving for harm.

There was science to support such orgasmic claims. Beverly Whipple and Barry Komisaruk, professors at Rutgers University, along with Gina Ogden of the Institute for Advanced Study of Human Sexuality, had collaborated in measuring the increased heart rate, blood pressure, pupil diameter, and tolerance for pain during orgasm in women who said they could come—without any touch at all—by imagining lovers or phrases of music. In the lab, the women were strapped to monitors. They rested their chins on an ophthalmology platform and stared through the eyepieces of a pupillometer. Then they made themselves climax both merely by thinking and by stroking their clitorises. No matter the method, the measurements were similar.

I wondered not only about the Baroness's orgasms but about the law governing how she got there. Was roasting someone on a spit legal? Did a submissive's consent mean that the sadist couldn't be prosecuted? In legal terms, could a person rationally agree to be assaulted, or was such willingness viewed as inherently irrational and legally void? The law was blurry. Probably the most relevant case involved a doctoral candidate in microbiology who, in the late 1990s, spent almost two years in prison for allegedly raping and burning, beating and biting a college student while keeping her roped to a futon for twenty hours. The conviction was eventually overturned on appeal, because the trial judge had refused to allow the jury to consider e-mail messages sent by the girl to the defendant laying out her masochistic desires. Consent, the ruling implied, couldn't be disregarded.

The S-M community had its own standards, its own principles. "Safe, sane, consensual" were the hallowed words. Neither the Baroness nor Master R had much use for them. "Safe is limiting," Master R said disdainfully. "And what is sanity?" Consent was just a beginning. He preferred to adhere to a different code, "the code of love." He loved his slaves, he said, and expounded on the meaning of the word, paraphrasing the philosopher George Santayana: "Love is a physical drive with an ideal intent."

AT dawn, after my night at Master R's, I walked outside to the spit, which remained, two years later, next to an untended vegetable garden, tomato and zucchini stalks from seasons ago softening to mulch beneath a riot of blackberry bushes. The sky was clearing fast, clouds skating toward oblivion. The gray steel immensity looked like one of Richard Serra's outdoor sculptures: hulking, incomprehensible. "That day had that wonderful incongruity," the Baroness had said. "The gorgeous autumn weather, the sun, the blue sky, and the next thing you know you're at the heart of darkness."

We drove back to the city. As we came close to Manhattan, the Baroness phoned her husband to say she was almost home. "Hello, handsome," she began adoringly, and the affection stayed in her voice throughout the conversation. She called again a half hour later to say she was very near. When we reached her building he was waiting there to kiss her and welcome her back.

THE Girl in her horse blinkers, Frank with his spiral notebook, Elvis on his spit—all were in important company. Jean-Jacques Rousseau spent his life yearning to replicate the whippings of his childhood governess but never, he wrote, "daring to declare my tastes." And in ancient Athens, in the marketplace, the philosopher Peregrinus Proteus masturbated while Athenians lashed him at his request. He later cremated himself at the Olympic Games of 165.

Richard von Krafft-Ebing, an Austro-German psychiatrist, coined the terms "sadism" and "masochism" in the late nineteenth century. Sadism he drew from the Marquis de Sade, the French aristocrat and author who, a century earlier, lived in an ecstasy of assaulting women—slicing, poisoning, whipping—and lived often, too, in prison or a lunatic asylum. "Sex without pain," he said, "is like food without taste." Krafft-Ebing derived masochism from Baron Leopold von Sacher-Masoch, the nineteenth-century author of *Venus in Furs*, an autobiographical novel of submission that some of the Baroness's acolytes treated as a bible.

"A differentiation of original and acquired cases of sadism is scarcely possible," Krafft-Ebing wrote. "Many individuals, tainted from birth, for a long time do everything to conquer the perverse instinct. . . . Later, when the opposing motives of an ethical and aesthetic kind have been gradually overcome, and when oft-repeated experience has proved the natural act to give but incomplete satisfaction, the abnormal instinct suddenly bursts forth. Owing to this late expression, in acts, of an originally perverse disposition, the appearances are those of an acquired perversion. As a rule, it may be safely assumed that this psychopathic state exists from birth." He believed the same about masochism and most other erotic deviance: the conditions were inborn. And in *Psychopathia Sexualis* he recounted hundreds of case histories of the afflicted.

"Case 21. Vincenz Verzeni, born 1849: 'I had an unspeakable delight in strangling women, experiencing during the act erections and real sexual pleasure. . . . The feeling of pleasure while strangling them was much greater than that which I experienced while masturbating.'"

"Case 28. In the 60s the inhabitants of Leipzig were frightened by a man who was accustomed to attack young girls on the street, stabbing them in the upper arm with a dagger. Finally arrested, he was recognized as a sadist, who at the instant of stabbing had an ejaculation, and with whom the wounding of the girls was an equivalent for coitus."

"Case 57. 'I am thirty-five years old, mentally and physically normal. . . . Even in my early childhood I loved to revel in ideas about the absolute mastery of one man over others. . . . In reading *Uncle Tom's Cabin* (which I read about the beginning of puberty), I had erections. Particularly exciting for me was the thought of a man being hitched to a wagon in which another man sat with a whip, driving and whipping him.'"

Krafft-Ebing's heir, Magnus Hirschfeld, a German physician whose library on sexuality was burned by the Nazis, collected cases of deviance in a similar way. But with the desire to give or absorb pain and degradation, Hirschfeld saw an impulse so widespread that the word "deviance" couldn't fairly be applied. Soon after his death, his students put together a book of his teaching, *Sexual Anomalies*: "In the seventeenth and eighteenth centuries the flagellomania of Englishwomen became a sort of epidemic. One of the most remarkable manifestations of this tendency was the formation of female flagellation clubs, whose members were recruited exclusively from the upper classes." The women would meet one evening each week, much as a book club might, to whip each other, and brothels specializing in whippings were a popular and even accepted part of London life.

To read Krafft-Ebing and Hirschfeld between spending time with the Baroness was to see her within a long history but also to understand her rarity. Both scientists suggested that female masochism was common enough. But true female sadism was so hard to find that Krafft-Ebing, for all his avid assembling, related only two cases in *Psychopathia Sexualis*, both of women whose erotic charge came in sucking their husbands' blood. Krafft-Ebing and Hirschfeld included any number of prostitutes adept with whips and wives implored to enact scenes of punishment, but there was no woman to match Sacher-Masoch's ideal lover, the fictionalized master of *Venus in Furs*, who was compelled by her own desire.

The Baroness would have stood out in Krafft-Ebing's and Hirschfeld's research, as she did now in the night world of New York. There was no shortage of professionals. To type in "dominatrix Manhattan" on Google's search engine was to find Mistress Troy and Mistress Elizabeth and Mistress

Rebecca. It was to read about a mistress who specialized in "kidnapping and abduction" and "full toilet training," and another, Mz. Black Mistress, who declared, "I will confiscate your worthless nuts when you bow down to me baby." There were hundreds and maybe thousands of others who made or supplemented their living by supplying customers with subjection at an hourly rate, but, except possibly in a broad psychological sense, there was no sign of their taking pleasure. Some of them attended the monthly parties the Baroness threw at a bar near her shop: a tall, knife-bodied black woman; a pygmy-sized white woman whose makeup was pale as plaster; an art student with multicolored hair who hoped to find customers to help pay her tuition. They laughed as they gave out their floggings. They spat derision and condemnation as they flailed away with studded paddles, causing not only flesh but spines to shudder. They smiled as they ground their spiked heels into the testicles of men who lay beneath them. And perhaps they took satisfaction in having such power over the gender that, as a rule, had more. But they didn't speak of pleasure the way the Baroness did. They didn't speak of lips swelling. They didn't talk of protracted orgasms. They didn't talk, as the Baroness did when she remembered Genevieve or another slave, a man she'd named Luminous, about a transcendent connection, about a mutual desire so strong that sadist and masochist couldn't keep themselves away from each other; they didn't talk about being desperate and destined for each other; they didn't talk in terms of *each other*. They didn't speak—didn't come close to speaking—about being in the thrall of love.

The Baroness was a true female paraphiliac. There weren't many, except in the realm of masochism. In all the other categories, from acrotomophilia to zoophilia, women were, according to every sexologist I talked with, drastically underrepresented.

Some estimated the imbalance at ten to one. Most refused to estimate; the statistics just weren't there. But no one doubted the disproportion.

One theory, at least with the paraphilias that centered on body parts rather than sexual acts—on feet, say, as opposed to floggings—was that male desire arose much more from the visual, and so it was more vulnerable to misdirection. The theory was frequently linked to the idea of imprinting. In 1935, the Austrian zoologist Konrad Lorenz had performed an experiment. As a brood of goslings hatched, he made sure that he, and not the mother goose, was the first being the hatchlings saw. The goslings, who would normally have followed their mother everywhere, instead followed Lorenz. He had successfully become their mother by presenting himself during the brief window when the goslings' brains were innately programmed to take in and store their mother's identity, to be imprinted with this information. Some sexologists believed that similar factors might be at work with the particulars of male desire, that during boyhood periods when certain hormonal surges occur, surges that may be momentary or protracted and that come most likely before puberty, the brain is open to imprinting that then defines erotic attraction. A boy's endocrine and neurological systems are intertwined so that, at these susceptible times, his erotic ideals become fixed in the brain. The times for imprinting may not be as limited as the goslings'—a few seconds or minutes don't necessarily determine the direction of eros. No proponent of the theory was sure about the windows of susceptibility, or about all the hormones involved, or about the mechanism of imprinting. When it came to desire, few sexologists were sure about anything.

And such theorizing didn't fully address the question of why women are so rarely paraphilic—or address the problem of how female desire finds its direction. Meredith Chivers, a psychologist in Toronto, had chosen to devote her young career to these unknowns.

In her lab, in a faceless concrete building belonging to one of Canada's most important psychiatric teaching hospitals, on a floor of sexuality researchers where she was the only woman, she wore narrow, stylish rectangular glasses and graceful black boots that laced up almost to her knees. Her blond hair fell over a low-necked black top.

She joked that she'd been studying sex since the age of five, when she first contemplated the reasons for kissing: "I was sitting next to my mom in our family's giant Chevrolet Impala station wagon, and feeling very small—cars have always made me feel small—and my five-year-old brain was chugging away. Why would they do this, why would people kiss? My parents weren't kissing at that moment, but I'd seen them, and I'd seen other people, and I wanted to know why this would occur. We were pulling out from our compound of townhouses onto Three Valleys Drive. It's bizarre to me that I remember this one event in such detail. As we were going over the curb, right at that instant, the thought suddenly went through my head: *That's* why they do it; men and women kiss because they're going to have babies."

Twenty-eight years later she was not only alone as a woman among her colleagues but alone in studying female eros. When she'd first arrived on the floor of sexologists, Kurt Freund was still alive and doing research there. She asked why he never studied women.

Half a century earlier, in Czechoslovakia, Freund had been employed by the Czech military to help catch conscripts who were trying to evade service by pretending to be homosexual. He developed a mechanism, called a plethysmograph, to quantify male arousal to various stimuli. A glass tube was placed over the penis, with an airtight seal around the base of the shaft. Images were shown. A gauge detecting increases in air pressure measured the swelling of the organ. If the air pressure didn't rise when Freund showed erotic slides of young men, the conscript was headed into the army.

Freund was, meanwhile, among the first modern-era psychiatrists to argue that homosexuality arose from prenatal biology rather than childhood experience, and that it could not be treated. At the start of his career, he had tried to cure gays through psychoanalysis; eventually he called in his patients and gave back their money. He worked to repeal Czech laws that criminalized gay sex, and later, after he'd fled Communist rule and settled in Toronto, his understanding of homosexuality as permanent and harmless helped to convince the American Psychiatric Association, in 1973, to remove the orientation from its list of psychiatric disorders.

Bald, with big ears and a nose like a scythe, Freund answered Chivers's question with his own: "How am I to understand what it is to be a woman? Who am I to study women when I'm a man?" And in his words she heard an affirmation of what she suspected, that when it came to the workings of erotic attraction men and women might be entirely different.

She knew of an unpublished study showing that the degree of genital arousal in heterosexual women watching videos of heterosexual and lesbian sex was "undifferentiated." The women, Chivers said, "were responding to everything." In a series of studies of her own, she replicated this result and added other stimuli, including a video featuring the copulation of bonobos, a species of ape closely related to the chimpanzee. She made the bonobo movie herself, finding footage of bonobo sex. Because the soundtrack was insufficient ("bonobos don't seem to make much noise in sex, though the females give a kind of pleasure grin and make chirpy sounds"), she dubbed in some animated screeching. She led both women and men, heterosexual and homosexual, into her lab to watch and listen.

The lab consisted of two small rooms. One held a brown leatherette La-Z-Boy chair, a small TV sitting on a table, and, depending on the subject, a penile plethysmograph or the bulb and wires of the vaginal model. The bulb was long and slender, about a quarter-inch in diameter, with a broad stopper at the base to prevent it from slipping in too far. The light from the bulb was reflected off the vaginal walls; a photocell measured the reflection. The greater the flow of blood to the genitals, the more light bounced back. On a computer in the adjoining room, Chivers controlled the videos and monitored the subject's level of physiological arousal.

As the bonobos humped, blood ran to the women's vaginas. It didn't take long; physiological excitement was immediate, just as it was—no matter what the female subject's sexual orientation—when the screen showed women going down on women, men going down on men, men screwing men, and men copulating with women. The male subjects, though, grew physically aroused mostly in categorical ways: straight males responded to images of lesbian or heterosexual sex, gay males to scenes involving men. And the male subjects were unexcited by the apes.

After each film, a question popped up on the subject's screen: "How sexually aroused do you feel right now?" The subject replied on a keypad. The males answered in ways that corresponded to the measures of the plethysmograph. Their minds and penises, their subjective and objective scores, were in agreement. The females replied in ways that were much less related to the responses of their vaginas. They reported no immediate arousal to bonobo sex. To lesbian scenes, heterosexual women reported less excitement than their genitals indicated, to scenes of gay men they reported a great deal less, and to heterosexual scenes they reported much more. For women, all seemed confusion. Adding to the muddle, Chivers pondered a study demonstrating women's arousal to sexual assault, and a report showing that some women reach orgasm during rape. Her own experience as a clinician confirmed this.

The muddle, she believed, might be due to thinking about female sexuality in male terms. Men's genitals responded to specific categories of stimuli, and these responses matched their psychological desires: if this was *the* standard, then women were a mess. But what if it was only *a* standard? What if, for women, physical readiness for sex was distinct from the lust for it? What if there was another legitimate system of desire?

"I feel like a pioneer on the edge of a giant forest," Chivers said. Between stints in Toronto, she'd done another version of her obsessive research, while working under Michael Bailey, a renowned sexologist at Northwestern University in Chicago. Looking at Chivers's data showing swift vaginal engorgement to images of all sorts of human sexual activity, Bailey had suggested that women are inherently bisexual, but Chivers had balked at this idea. It seemed to apply a male paradigm— heterosexual, homosexual, bisexual—to something deeply unknown. "I do think that for women preferences exist," she told me. "Women do choose to have sex with men or with women or with both. But I don't know if it happens for the same reasons men seek out partners. I don't know that it's driven by a sexually motivated system, by sexual desire in and of itself. Is there a basic sexual rudder for women?" she asked, and said that she suspected there might not be, that "emotional kindling" might prove to be far more important in the erotic directions women took.

There was an "interesting relationship," she wrote to me later, describing the work of another researcher, "between sex drive and attraction to same-sex or opposite-sex people. As sex drive becomes stronger in men, their attractions to men and women are more polarized. Women, however, show greater sexual attraction to both women and men as sex drive gets stronger. This suggests that sex drive is working in concert with a mechanism in men to direct sexuality toward one gender or another, whereas in women this mechanism may not exist and therefore greater sex drive is expressed with both genders."

"There's this gravity," she said, "in the academic world, to look at male and female sexuality from the perspective of equality, of sameness. Any indicators of difference are seen as socially constructed—or else the methodology of the research is seen as flawed. I feel like I'm going to fight an uphill battle in saying, 'No, male and female sexuality are really different, and you're going to have to look at them differently.'"

She didn't know what she would find in the forest. The genital arousal to assault she and others saw as self-protection; in evolutionary terms, prehistoric women had needed to be vaginally receptive to sexual aggression in order to avoid laceration and tearing. Perhaps female responsiveness to bonobo sex was related to this. Perhaps the sight of an erect penis was all it took to stir this primordial system of self-preservation. But then why the physiological arousal to lesbian scenes, an arousal more powerful than to scenes of homosexual men? And why—as she added videos—the arousal to a lone naked woman more than to a solitary nude man? And what would happen if she replaced the apes with chickens? How closely did the sexual participants have to resemble humans? What exactly were the women responding to?

Young though she was, Chivers knew that a lifetime of research might take her barely inside the forest's edge, might allow her only a dim glimpse of the factors that shaped female desire. "One of the things I think about," she said, "is the diad formed by men and women. Certainly women are very sexual and have the capacity to be even more sexual than men, but one possibility is that instead of it being a go-out-and-get-it kind of sexuality it's more of a reactive process. If you have this diad, and one part is pumped full of testosterone, is more interested in risk-taking, is probably a bit more aggressive, you've got a very strong motivational force. It wouldn't make sense to have another similar force. You need something complementary. And I've often thought that there is something really powerful for women's sexuality about being desired. That receptivity element. At some point I'd love to do a study that would look at that. We just don't know much about it right now."

On her floor of sexologists, Chivers was surrounded by men studying paraphilias, and she wondered if the scarcity of female deviants was the result of male definitions. If the system for women was fundamentally different, then the paraphilias would be different as well. They wouldn't be on the existing list. For women, the map of the typical and the aberrant hadn't yet been drawn. The mapmaker would have to work her way through the giant forest. But in terms of traditionally defined paraphilias, it made sense to her that women seemed most likely to be masochists. Flesh bared and waiting for the whip, or limbs bound, or body suspended from the ceiling, the masochist was desired, receptive, the focus of the sadist's lustful gaze.

Chivers knew that women might be undercounted among

traditional paraphiliacs. The man who flashed his erection at a toll booth would be arrested and perhaps treated for exhibitionism; the woman who flashed her breasts would more likely win applause. The expectations and allowances of the culture might be distorting the numbers. And she knew that the forces of culture might be affecting her own research. Physiological arousal to wide-ranging stimuli might be, as Freud had argued, the natural state for both males and females. Was it simply that the culture taught men more emphatically to restrict their lust to limited sets of targets while female desire was allowed more freedom? Was it merely that men, having internalized these lessons at the deepest level, responded physically within categories that were learned rather than natural? Were men and women different primarily because of experience rather than the innate? Chivers and her husband, Michael Seto, one of the researchers on her floor, talked about someday attempting an experiment that would use a type of magnetic resonance imaging to test whether particular inhibitory regions of the brain were more active in males than females as a variety of erotic stimuli were shown. And Chivers had already tried to eliminate learned inhibition as an explanation of her results. She had included male-to-female transsexuals among her subjects. These medically created women, both those who were heterosexual and those who were homosexual, showed categorical response patterns. They responded like men. This seemed to point to a system that was inborn. Yet one could argue that the forces of culture, of learning, had taken permanent hold within these subjects long before their surgeries and their emergence as females could have shifted the culture's input. Chivers couldn't fully isolate the innate, knew she might never be able to. The forest often looked impenetrable.

But one thing was almost certain: women like the Baroness were nearly alone.

And for much of her life, feeling a difference she could not identify, she had wanted to die.

AROUND the time of our trip to Master R's, the Baroness heard a Latin phrase. She had left school at thirteen. Now she listened to Proust on tape, was proud of her self-education, and was enamored, right away, of the words *sui generis*. The phrase means "of its own kind." She felt this described her perfectly, felt she had been generated as though out of air. The hardships of her growing up, she insisted, had little or nothing to do with who she had become. They couldn't explain her style or power or sexuality. "I am *sui generis*," she said, elated, then paused in contemplation. "Yes. I like that."

She'd grown up in group homes and small orphanages in Britain until she was twelve. "There was nothing really horrible going on. The cruelest thing I remember is having to eat Spam, throwing up, and being made to continue eating it." Much of her time had been taken up by reading. She'd been captivated by a series of books called *The Famous Five*: four kids and a dog hunting treasure and tracking down thieves. She wrote her own version. "It was a compilation of all the kids in one character. There was no damned dog, not even a cat. She was orphaned at a young age, free and independent, and I took my book around to the neighbors to sell."

At twelve she was adopted; her new parents soon moved with her to the States, to Los Angeles. At thirteen she began running away repeatedly. She spent long stretches of her teenage years in San Francisco during the sixties. "This is how I remember that period. I was awake and muttering for days at a time. I was frightened of people. The police picked me up off the street. If you'd told me there was something about me that was fabulous, I certainly wouldn't have believed it. I had suicide headaches. For two or three years I saw only in black-and-white. I had shock treatments. Two times? Three times? Thirteen or fourteen would have been the first one. I feel I deserve everything I have now because I paid for it.

"I remember being happy for the first time. There are moments when you know you're truly happy. I'd just taken about sixty Seconal, and I thought I'd succeeded. But then I didn't die. Some of this stuff is so embarrassing. I went down a tunnel. It's so clichéd, and the last thing I want to be is common. There was a white light at the end, a triangle glowing white, and a conversation with some sort of being, invisible, at the center. Basically I was told that I couldn't leave because I hadn't realized my purpose in life. I said, 'Tell me what it is. I'll do it, and I'll be right back.' And the voice said, 'No, you have to find out.' And I felt myself being pulled back out through the tunnel."

Decades passed, decades of too many drugs, decades of designing costumes for movies and the theater (she had taught herself to sew at one of the British orphanages, and in San Francisco as a teenager she had made clothing and sold it on the streets), blurred decades of incidents impossible for her to place in time, partly, she felt, because the electroshock treatments had damaged her hold on chronology, but partly, too, it seemed, because an indifference to time fit with her sense of who she was and how she'd become herself—*sui generis*—with feeling that she had simply arisen. In the mid-seventies she moved to Manhattan. Two decades later, at a birthday party of hers—her birthday was on Halloween—a guest arrived dressed in rubber and carrying a bullwhip. He held out the whip toward her.

By that point she'd been married to Mark for almost ten years and with him for thirteen. They'd met at Chemical Bank's headquarters, where he was a corporate photographer. He'd just moved to New York from Wisconsin, where he'd grown up as the son of a man who built water-softening machines and sold them himself across the Midwest. Her boyfriend at the time, who worked in Mark's department, stood her up for lunch one day. She had come to the office wearing "the most conservative clothes she could put together," Mark remembered. "A white blouse with big sleeves, a huge collar, a short white skirt. Far from corporate."

They were drawn to each other right away, he to her boldness, to a woman he called "the only person I've ever met who is completely unfettered by convention," and she to his stability, to a man she saw as "my rock." Knowing her affection for the thirties and forties, he proposed to her at the Rainbow Room, between dances to the swing band, and they honeymooned in Paris, where he discovered his love for taking pictures of dogs. He began with a beagle that he noticed trying to drink from a bottle of beer. Soon he was photographing pugs and labs and dachshunds in adorable poses, tongues out, ears cocked, eyes plaintive, heads tilted fetchingly. "We are passionate about pets," his Web site would later announce. "And we love nothing more than finding and capturing the unique character of each one we meet."

After their honeymoon, they settled down in the East Village. Their erotic life was traditional, with a coil of desire tightened by the months when she traveled to make costumes for films and they were apart. Then, at her Halloween birthday party, the guest offered his whip.

"I believe I literally took several steps backward. I put up a barrier. I knew it—I knew that if I touched it I would be doomed. Nothing happened that night. But we got to know each other. I carved a V into his back shortly afterward. With a pin, but I do mean carved as opposed to scratched. With a fair amount of blood. We learned a lot together, he and I. It was on his body that I learned to use a whip the way it should be used. It's one of the ways that I'm a geek. I like to do something over and over until I'm good at it. It should feel like touching."

Early in her education, her birthday guest, whom she later named Luminous, took her to the city's best-known S-M club. What she lacked, then, in skill, she made up for in unrestrained lust. "Everyone is going to be talking about you," her partner promised at the end of the evening. About "safe, sane, consensual," she made it plain from the start that she didn't observe rules.

Before Luminous arrived in her life, she'd had some inkling of her unconventional yearnings. She remembered excitement, long ago, as she'd watched an old black-and-white movie: a British sailor bound to the mast and flogged. After his arrival, she felt she had found out something central about herself and, in expressing what had lain dormant for so long, that she "became a more balanced person, a nicer person." And the question of purpose, posed by the voice within the white triangle, was answered. "I can give people their dreams. I have the power to change people. I get to do so much good." She could liberate "the core of being" in the city's masochists just as her own sadism had been freed. She could save them from the unhappiness and self-destruction that had besieged so much of her life. She could be, she said, "a beacon" to people like the Girl and Frank and Genevieve and Elvis and the countless others she had lured into confronting their desires for the first time or into receiving what they had needed.

The clothing she designed was part of her plan to unbury

the erotic truth in those who had endured thwarted lives. She saw the city as filled with women and men waiting, consciously or unconsciously, for such unburying. They were like homosexuals who suppressed their desire and distorted or destroyed the rest of themselves as well. The same was true for the masochist. The same had been true for her. She envisioned a multiplying flock finding their way to her, and the latex was one of the ways she pulled them in. The lubrication of the body that was required to slide the garment over the skin; the sudden encasement; the immaculate smoothness of this second flesh; its gleam, for she had her submissives shine every item in the boutique; the material's capacity to create something sleek from the contours of any person of any shape; the way the wearer's nerve endings responded if so much as the back of a fingernail was dragged lightly over the surface, a response somehow twice as electric as if the same gesture was carried out directly upon the skin—before anything explicit had transpired, her customers were already in a state of partial surrender.

OUTSIDE New York's annual Black and Blue Ball, the sidewalk and street were thronged with guests and onlookers, photographers, security guards. When the Baroness emerged from a taxi with Lara on a braided rubber leash hooked to a collar, it seemed that everyone coalesced. The Baroness wore a floor-length gown of amethyst-colored latex with a pattern of ruffles cascading down the back and a train that Lara lifted off the pavement. Cameras flashed and people called out to her and someone from the ball's staff guided her away from the main line and directly toward the door.

Inside, amid the crush of men in top hats and tails and women in black wigs and rubber corsets and men naked but for leather jock straps and women clothed only in thin leather bands, guests paid homage to the Baroness. The loud pulse of dance music made their words difficult to hear, but again and again, on all fours, they kissed the toes or heels of her shoes or, heads bent and bodies bowed, pressed their lips to the back of her hand. It didn't matter if they were leashed to another master. White men being led by black women; bare-chested women crawling alongside male owners or female dominatrixes—they showed their reverence for the Baroness without objection from those controlling them.

The ball was less an occasion for play than a yearly convocation and night of greeting. Up on the brass-railed balcony above the dance floor, the Baroness ran into David, who approached her without any gesture of deference. Once, they had tried to develop a way of talking with their whips, each on separate rooftops; they had imagined a Morse code of whip-cracking. His face was haggard and, in a tank top, his arms were like wires—he had AIDS—but he could stand in the middle of Union Square Park and make the windows of the surrounding buildings, sixty yards away, rattle as the end of his whip broke the sound barrier.

Below the balcony, an MC interrupted the dancing to announce that Carrie, one half of the lesbian couple that hosted the ball, had just given birth to a baby boy. David drifted away and Eliza and Ben drifted over.

They were long and narrow, with dark hair and faces that seemed to belong on the covers of magazines. She worked as a fund-raiser, he as an architect. Sheathed in the Baroness's latex, Eliza in red, Ben in black, she wearing six-inch heels and he platform boots, they might have been a pair of cartoon heroes ready to kick their way through animated adventures. But their adventures were erotic.

Eliza hadn't always looked so arresting, not in this way. She'd had childhood arthritis. She'd used a walker and crutches and a cane through adolescence, spent her summers at a place she called "cripple camp," endured her own terrifying oddity growing up in the Maine town where her father owned a hardware store. "I felt no control over my body," she remembered the years of illness that hadn't ended until her late teens or early twenties. "I was sick, the pain was constant, and this is part of what that did to me: I don't want to be powerless; how can I have power? This is one way to experiment with that. There are times when I'm totally dominant. But there are other times when I'm completely submissive. I want that intimacy, that pain. I want to feel: I've been here before but not like this."

I've been here before but not like this—her words echoed the psychological theory that we eroticize what has frightened us, shamed us, wounded us. In this way we attempt to escape our deepest hurt and confusion. Eliza didn't dismiss explanations the way the Baroness did. She saw her arthritis as central to her sexuality, not only because it had made her long for both power and pain but because the strangeness of her young body and the alienation it had caused her made it easier to embrace difference now. She sought it out. And when she thought of her friends from cripple camp there seemed a high percentage who later found themselves on alternate sexual paths.

Ben couldn't conjure explanations, only early beginnings: the basement game he'd devised for himself and his neighborhood friends at the age of four or five, ending always with his imprisonment in an old unused diaper bin; the game in the woods at the age of twelve or thirteen, culminating with his being tied to a tree and two or three girls jabbing him with sticks.

Through his twenties he'd been in love with a documentary filmmaker. "She was very liberal politically but personally very conservative." He'd endured their vanilla sex life by spending his early morning hours staring at S-M Web sites. A chance meeting with a professional dominatrix, a Japanese woman who was a graphic designer by day, pulled him past fantasy. He booked a session at the dungeon where she worked.

"The Baroness will call bullshit on all professionals," he said. "For her it's a purely human relationship. But they do offer an opportunity for guys who have this predilection, guys who are driven crazy, guys who are just, like, I really want to figure out who I am."

The session with the graphic designer helped Ben in the figuring out, and by the time he met Eliza at a bar, his yearning leaped out in the first flirtation. "If I have to have vanilla sex one more time," he told her, "I'm going to shoot myself." Without knowing exactly what he meant, she sensed he was what she needed. She'd been dating a man who wanted to marry her, and whom she couldn't love because of something she felt missing in bed between them.

Now they spent their nights and weekends at play with each other. "When we first got together we were two subs," he said. "Clearly someone's got to top. And once we started doing it, it expanded our experience." This kind of versatility, too, the Baroness held in some disdain. But one recent evening he had burned thirty welts into Eliza's buttocks with a cigarette. On another night he had come as, lightly, she whipped his penis. "It was so demeaning and so hot," he said.

To be the one in control was far more demanding. "You might commit yourself to carrying out a certain form of bondage," he explained. "And then you think, I want to do *that*, but now she is all tied up this way and in order to get there I have to get her out, and it becomes inorganic. You want everything to flow. It requires choreographing. Like throwing a dinner party: come in, how are you, let me take your coat, sit down, something to drink. But if you walk in and right away there's a three-course meal sitting in front of you and it's only six-thirty: no. Things have to make sense next to each other, to emerge from each other."

"Sometimes it's seamless," she said, "and sometimes it's, Oh fuck oh shit."

"We forgive each other."

"I love being in a relationship where I care about Ben to the nth degree."

Lately they had begun wounding and debasing each other in public, at parties thrown by friends they'd met at clubs or through the Baroness. "We love the public degradation of it. The audience adds to the humiliation." So going to parties meant packing gear: "The first few times, it was like we needed a checklist. Clothespins. Ankle restraints. Wrist restraints. Ball weights. Leash. Collar. Gag. Masks. Opera-length rubber gloves. Carabiners. Flogger. Whip. Lighter. Locks. Keys. It's great to go fetish-shopping at Home Depot. Three sets of keys each for six regular and four mini locks—one set on a rubber band around the wrist, another set in the bag, another in a coat pocket. You don't want the love of your life chained up and no way to release her at the end of the night. All that equipment and you're decked in latex and then, 'Shit, we forgot cigarettes,' and we can't go into our corner deli looking like that. But all the preparation is worth it. The humiliation is so sensual."

Their play, their lovemaking, could go on for hours and hours. Still, when it was all over, when the submissive had stopped crying out in abject ecstasy, recovery wasn't as difficult as it might seem. "There's a feeling of complete exhaustion and exhilaration," she said. "It's not like I have to crawl out of a hole that's six feet under." And he: "I just curl up in her lap."

They had a saying, a vow they'd taken: "Everything always." Not with anyone else—they were faithful to each other—but between themselves. And not if it meant exposure within their other lives. They feared for her job if anyone at her organization found out. They feared for his commissions. People might be intrigued, might feel a tremor of self-recognition, that they possessed at least an element of similar yearning. But few would admit it. Most would react badly. Most wouldn't want them around. Even in downtown Manhattan, where they lived, they rarely walked outside for any distance in their latex, out of worry that the clothes would give them away to strangers on the street.

They felt that the Baroness truly was, for them and even more for the many others who were more secretive, more fearful, a beacon. The name she'd given herself, the boutique she owned, the way she appeared every day and night on the streets of Manhattan—Eliza and Ben saw her as a herald for the gift that, despite their fears, they felt lucky to have received. "It is difficult to live this way," he said. "There are social obstacles. But if someone said, 'I can take care of this perversion, you won't even miss it'—no way. This brings us too much. We wouldn't trade this for the world."

"PEOPLE don't believe it's an equal partnership," Mark said of his marriage to the Baroness. "They assume I play the role of a submissive."

He didn't, he told me. He had fallen in love with a woman with another name; he had married a woman who showed no signs of what she would become. The first time she used a whip he was stunned. It was in their living room, with Luminous, who had once been the highest-ranked chess player in the state of Arkansas, receiving her lashes. It was difficult for Mark to watch, to realize "that the woman I love has an interest in treating people this way. But it also seemed like a fluke, like it would be just that once. Had I known it was the start of a trend maybe I would have said something. Every year she seemed to enjoy inflicting a little more pain, taking a little more blood." He remembered his jealousy when she'd carved the V into Luminous's back. It had seemed so intimate.

She was his when it came to conventional sex. And gradually he had come to terms with her needing something more. "I think of it as two aspects of the woman I love. If she enjoys dispensing pain and humiliation, I'm glad that there is someone to take it. I have zero interest. I'm an outsider in her world. I've become acclimated. But I have no real friends in the S-M scene because *that* is what they have in common. It is still foreign to me. I still don't understand it. The more equal I feel with someone, the closer I feel."

ONE evening the Baroness invited me to drinks with her oldest friend. She had known Celeste for almost twenty-five years, since they'd met while working on costumes for a Broadway musical. At the quiet wine bar where we talked, Celeste wore black pants, a lavender cardigan, a necklace of small glass balls. Her voice was as delicate as the glass. Her brown hair was cropped short in the aftermath of cancer treatments that had accomplished what they could. She had a brain tumor; she was dying.

"The Baroness and Mark were the second people I told." She talked about her years of friendship with the Baroness, years of going to plays and the opera. And she talked about the Baroness's recent loyalty, her frequent visits, her willingness not to turn away from weakness and death. Celeste mentioned, too, that the Baroness had dispatched one of her submissives to help her with chores around her apartment. "I wouldn't have gotten through it without this woman sitting here as my friend."

"She has a brain tumor, she can't be trusted," the Baroness said, smiling, deflecting some of the sentiment.

Then Celeste said abruptly, "I'm not sure I'm over the shock yet. She was, before, extremely antiviolence. She couldn't even stand it if I got angry. She hits people. She hurts people. I was really, really shocked to see what she was doing to Luminous; it made me want to throw up. There were times, after her change, when I thought I could not be her friend. She was cutting and branding him. I couldn't deal with that. It wasn't him specifically, it was that she was doing this to another human being."

The Baroness stiffened. Her metallic eye shadow did nothing to brighten her wounded eyes. The conflagration of her hair seemed to collapse, the colors fading.

"I saw Charles, who is black, chained and serving as a slave at her apartment," Celeste went on in her fragile voice. "And when I protested, she said, 'This is sexy.'"

"As it was."

"And she talks about liking intelligence in her slaves."

"As I do."

"But doesn't it get in the way of their intelligence when they cower in front of you?" Celeste turned from me to face her friend.

"All their potential is wasted until they become who they are."

"Don't you destroy intelligence by tearing people down?"

"Have I mentioned"—the Baroness glanced at me—"that she has a brain tumor and can't be trusted?"

They laughed together.

"It's scary," Celeste said. "She really is happier as the Baroness."

FOR her Valentine's night party the Baroness wore pink latex gauntlets that rose to her shoulders and a black latex dress with a high sheen. Her hair was sculpted into a flaming arch. It was early. The bar she and her flock took over on the first Sunday of every month wasn't half-full. Two middle-aged men, both in latex bodysuits, chatted about the routes they'd taken to reach here. One had come from Pennsylvania, the other from New Jersey, and they complained mildly about the weather and the traffic as they might have done if this were a holiday gathering and they were relatives with little else to discuss. They'd both wound up in the Holland Tunnel; they compared their luck in the different lanes they'd chosen.

Then they were distracted. A lithe woman in her early twenties had climbed up onto the small stage. She spoke to the Baroness, who sipped a cocktail. They walked over to a chair her submissives carried from her apartment each month on these occasions. It looked like an old-fashioned electric chair. Made of wood, it was large and sturdy, straight-backed and spare. The woman, curly blond hair cut short and wearing only an ivory-colored slip, knelt backward on the seat. The Baroness locked her wrists tightly to large screw eyes. The woman's neck hung over the back. Her ankles were soon immobilized, and her waist was pinned by heavy tape, wrapped round and round from waist to wood.

The Baroness stepped about twelve feet from the chair and used a backhanded technique. Each lash against the woman's shoulders brought a gasp, a cry. Then the Baroness set aside the whip to attach dozens of clothespins to the woman's neck and shoulders and arms, and a metal clip to her tongue, which now protruded unnaturally, painfully, from her mouth. After more lashes, one of the Baroness's submissives removed the clothespins. A chain of welts decorated the flesh. Someone raised the woman's slip to expose more skin, which, with more flogging, began to bleed.

The Baroness paused again. "I try to force myself to slow down, to make it last," she told me afterward. "Especially with someone like that who wants it so badly, so openly." She approached the woman and stroked her lightly under the chin and along the neck. The woman laid her head to the side, worshipful. Her clipped tongue lolled. Around it her mouth tried to smile. Her eyes gazed supplicatingly at the Baroness, who gazed back like a lover in the midst of intercourse, positioned on top, ceasing her thrusts to look tenderly, almost pityingly at her partner before bringing them both to climax.

She resumed, slowly at first and then, after a few lashes, more quickly, harder. The woman's lower back and buttocks were streaked red, and between the streaks the skin looked as though a bulb were shining from underneath; it glowed a dark, garish pink. The gasps and cries became agonized, sensual groans. The Baroness's eyes had a manic flatness, a half-seeing focus. The whip struck and struck. She was silent, in a trance.

Afterward she moved close again. I watched with Sam, who had recently begun to receive her lashings and whose wife had the ladder of scars that the Baroness adored. The Baroness placed her fingers on the wounds she'd just made. Her eyes were closed. She touched gently, almost without pressure, slowly shifting her fingertips. The heat from the damaged skin spread through her hand the way a child's fever floods the lips of a kissing mother. Her eyes remained peacefully shut. The woman was still. The fingertips traced the topography of lacerations. "That's the Baroness," Sam said. "She nurtures you."

THE WATER'S EDGE

PART III

THE WATER'S EDGE

AFTER HIS METAMORPHOSIS, ROY SAT, ONE MORNING each week, in a windowless room. It had a blue industrial carpet, a blackboard, a circle of brown cushioned office chairs. A faint hum came from the air ducts. To reach the room from the waiting area, on the second floor of the probation building, Roy and the other men walked down a series of corridors and around a series of turns that felt like a path through a maze. The room was wedged in a back corner.

Roy burrowed through his mind relentlessly, trying to unbury an explanation for his being here, in the circle of twelve chairs. It seemed to him that he'd been, just yesterday, a normal man, approaching forty. "I was typical," he told me plaintively. "Typical. With the same fantasies generally that general men have."

He'd run a crew of computer technicians, repairing telecommunications equipment for Wall Street trading firms. In his off hours he'd led a wedding band that played the Plaza. He sang Frank Sinatra and Barry White with such agility, such

precise and layered mimicry, that to listen to his CDs, the re-
cordings he'd once mailed out to the couples thinking of book-
ing him, was to mistake his versions for the real thing.

> *You'll never find*
> *As long as you live*
> *Someone who loves you*
> *Tender like I do*

Barry White's low, late-night croon slid from Roy's lips as
though the black balladeer inhabited him. Roy was, in a sense,
a failed musician. His career had peaked when he was a teenager; a song he'd written and recorded, an antidrug anthem
with a disco beat, was played a few times on one of New York
City's major radio stations. For his own music, that had been
the beginning and the end. But his imitative talent was so extreme as to be original. He was somehow not a failure at all.
His replications held an ineffable richness that belonged to the
known singers but that he, magically, owned. Something oth-
erworldly, a kind of emotional, artistic channeling, happened
when he sang.

In what time work and music allowed, Roy flew kites—kites
bigger than most living rooms. One was an airborne acoustic
guitar in bright yellow. Another was a floating box of Cray-
ola crayons. At night he launched a kite outfitted with strobe
lights that pulsed the colors of the rainbow over the earth below. To the gargantuan bodies he attached streamers and spin-
ners, spiked balls and "watermelon tails," jellyfish tentacles and
"space socks" that trailed more than a hundred feet behind. His
kites could perform ballets with him holding the lines.

In the aftermath of his metamorphosis, he could recall no
history of longing for young girls. He'd had no criminal record

of any kind. "Not even a speeding ticket," he said. His trans-formation, it seemed to him, had begun abruptly one summer, on vacation at the beach. His second wife had pointed out her eleven-year-old daughter's body. Roy and his wife were stand-ing on the sand; his stepdaughter, Faith, and her best friend, Elizabeth, played several yards in front of them at the edge of the surf. "Look at those girls," Roy remembered his wife saying. "They're changing already. You can see their bodies changing."

LIKE Nabokov's Humbert, he sometimes felt that his adult en-trancement had its seed in childhood desire. Everyone knows Humbert's Lolita but few remember his Annabelle, though she enters on page one, introduced to explain, at least partially, his later crimes. "In point of fact," Humbert says, linking his crav-ing for Lolita to the infatuation he'd felt, decades earlier, on the cusp of adolescence, "there might have been no Lolita at all had I not loved, one summer, a certain initial girl-child." The memory of his pubescent love, the still-palpable recollection of urgent, exquisite fondling in the garden while Annabelle's parents were inside playing cards, leaves him with a lifelong yearning to recapture that sweetness, that desperation, that in-tensity, and to consummate what youth had thwarted. Lolita, whom Humbert pursues in his late thirties, is the incarnation of erotic nostalgia.

Roy's Annabelle was his aunt, his mother's much younger sister, thirteen when Roy was eleven. One summer night, on vacation with his mother's family, while the adults played cards in the kitchen, his aunt asked him to come into the sun room. And there, evening by evening, they progressed from display-ing to touching to her straddling him, their groins bare. She slid and rubbed herself across his cock. "I think that's what was always in my head with Faith," he said. He'd longed to have again that trembling childhood thrill.

But the explanation didn't come close to satisfying him. His soft, smooth face and easy, band leader's smile often collapsed in confusion. He was round in the middle and broad in the shoulders—bearish in a way that was more panda-like than threatening. In the back room at the end of the maze, near him along the circle of chairs, sat an elderly man with a graceful wave of white hair combed back from his forehead. There was a well-scrubbed man in his mid-thirties, his forehead shiny, the pale blue check in his button-down shirt matching the blue of his eyes.

They were there for group counseling as part of their probation. They had spent time in jail or prison: a few weeks; several years. The man with the wave of white hair had fondled the vagina of his grandniece again and again when the girl was seven, eight. He'd kissed her chest, had her hold his penis. As an adult, David, the man in the checked shirt, had given a blow job to his eleven-year-old brother. Later, he'd taken his six-year-old daughter to a motel room along with his brother, who was by then sixteen. He'd grown obsessed by a fantasy. Now he started to make it real. He persuaded them both to undress. David urged his brother to have sex with his daughter, only desisting "seconds away from something really, really bad happening," when his brother began to cry.

"What possessed me?" Roy demanded over and over in the group sessions and alone with himself. The question churned through the minds of most of the men. David, a published poet, said he felt like Dr. Jekyll and Mr. Hyde.

"Could *anybody* end up getting into this mess?" Roy asked.

• • •

"BEGIN breathing slowly and deeply," Patrick Liddle, the group's therapist, its leader, instructed the men. It was the way he often started. They sat with their hands on their thighs, their eyes closed. "Inhale through your nose and exhale through your mouth." He taught them to meditate. He spoke in a soothing monotone, the voice he used with them always, no matter how disquieted, how uneasily self-aware their crimes made him feel. "Pay attention to your breath. Is each breath reaching down to your upper chest? Your lower chest? Your abdomen? Let the breathing deepen."

He was silent a long while, then resumed. "Focus your awareness in your feet. Just be aware of how they feel." Part of his job was to give the men ways to keep their lives under control, to keep themselves from transgressing again. The meditation was one method. "Now center your attention on the steady beating of your heart." Liddle wore fashionably tailored suits and shoes polished to a soft gloss. The clothes were part of the program. His boss set the dress code, to lend some measure of esteem to those in treatment, to elevate men who could hardly have fallen lower. For the therapists themselves, the clothes helped to lessen the taint of what they were dealing with.

"Picture in your mind a large open field covered in deep grass up to your waist. A light, warm breeze is blowing. Feel the breeze on your skin. Each thought that enters your mind becomes a brightly colored balloon; watch them float; just let them go." Roy and the others sat perfectly still. Their fingers curled gently. Their jaws were slack, their mouths slightly open. They seemed almost to be sleeping, and like sleeping men anywhere, they looked almost like children.

• • •

"NOW slowly open your eyes."

They returned from the field of tall grass to the faces of the others. Liddle sometimes asked them for introductions, though the faces stayed mostly the same. They went around the circle. "I was convicted of two counts of sexual assault four, and three counts of risk of injury to a minor, and enticing a minor over the Internet," Roy began. He forced himself not to mumble. Facing up to what he had done was a requirement for graduating from treatment. And he hoped this might lead—especially if he had Liddle's recommendation—to a judge's reducing his term of probation.

The treatment was grounded in an idea that seemed simple: to acknowledge both his crime and the anarchy of lust that lay within him was the first step toward his finding self-control. So the ability to confront himself, and to be candid with Liddle about his desires, was a requisite if he wanted to do anything outside the bounds of his probation restrictions: visit his parents over the state line, or go to a bowling alley or a movie or a family function, anyplace where he might come in contact with kids under sixteen. Any family gathering he attended had to be adults-only; he needed to leave right away if kids showed up. In his state, the group leaders and probation officers worked in tandem, weighing how well they could trust the men, and the therapists could be as cautious, as suspicious, as the probation officers. Together, Liddle and Roy's PO set the limits on his existence. And unless he got Liddle's recommendation and this led to a judge's mercy, it seemed Roy would be existing this way for the rest of his life.

"I was sentenced," he went on with his introduction, "to

twenty years suspended after thirty days, with thirty-five years probation. My offense behaviors I engaged in were touching my wife's daughter and her best friend sexually, touching them through their clothing between their legs, around their waist, moving my hand into the top of their waistband. I moved my hand under their shorts up to their panty lines. I used games that were called Chase and Spider to manipulate them into feeling safe with me." His voice lowered, sped up. He rushed on into the next part, into the online messages he'd sent to Faith, suggesting what they might do.

HE told me his story time and again, in detail he withheld from the group, as we sat at his kitchen table or in an empty conference room at his job. He was still a supervisor at the telecommunications repair company. In a squat suburban building just off a highway, at worktables in vast, orderly rooms, he and his team leaned over high-tech consoles and microprocessors with multicolored flashing diodes. They fixed the circuitry or, depending on Roy's decision, redesigned it. With the permission of Liddle and the probation department, he was allowed to work around computers as long as he never went online outside the watch of a colleague.

Everyone at his job was aware of his crime. He'd made a point of being open, of answering questions. The company's owner, who'd hired Roy several years ago, had testified on his behalf at his sentencing. "You're talking about a person I know," the owner told me. "A stranger, I would write them off, I wouldn't talk to them, I wouldn't see them, if they did one-tenth of what he did." And for Roy, within the squat building, it wasn't only the owner who forgave him. As I drove with him to work one winter morning, he said that he was engaged to be married again—to a bookkeeper at the company, a colleague since before his arrest. A few weeks earlier, at a Christmas Eve dinner at his house, he'd hidden a ring in the chocolate cake he served for dessert.

"THEY'RE starting to develop. Look at their behinds. Look at my daughter, how pretty she's going to be when she grows up." Telling me about his crime at the well-polished kitchen table in his neatly kept wooden house, he always began with the words of Faith's mother, Jackie, at the beach. "I'm going to have problems with her when she grows up. Sexually. With boys. I know I'm going to have a problem with her."

"Yeah," he said. "Look at you."

"Please. If she ends up like me I'm going to have to shoot myself."

He'd known Faith and her older brother from the time they were born. Their father had been a friend of Roy's since kindergarten and, for years, a member of Roy's band, until Jackie left him for Roy when the kids were around four and six. Roy had no children of his own. Faith and her brother lived with their father, but they spent lots of time at the house Roy shared with their mother. The boy, a prodigy on the drums, jammed in the basement with Roy on guitar. The time Roy spent with Faith was more childlike. But after that vacation at the shore, the games they played—often with her best friend, Elizabeth, too—grew sexualized at some level within his mind.

During Chase, he and the girls would turn off most of the lights. They plugged in a strobe light from his band equipment or a lamp that cast the shapes of moons on the walls, in blues and yellows and greens. His marriage was starting to come apart. Sometimes his wife was home, having shut herself in their bedroom for the evening. Sometimes she was out on her own. He raced after the girls through the house, through the colored beams.

"I remember times they would want to play Chase with me. I'd be sitting on the couch on Friday night, watching TV. I didn't want to play with them. I was beat. And they'd come pulling on me. They were the ones that talked me into it. And I remember they'd go into their room and put their bathing suits on. I never told them to do that. And they're running around the house shaking their butts at me."

In Spider, each player had to sit motionless; if you moved at all you got pinched. The touching occurred during both games, and the dutiful confession Roy delivered to the group implied that the touching was blatantly, consciously sexual on his part. But the truth, he felt, was more complex, more elusive. He believed that a change had occurred with Jackie's words on the beach, that he'd never before seen his stepdaughter as sexual, that a new awareness had penetrated at that moment, but he wasn't at all certain that his own thinking, during the games, was permeated by desire.

He was obsessively introspective about all that had happened. He thought back to his anger at his wife, his fleeting idea that if she was going to leave him taking care of her kids, then he was "going to get something out of this, too." Yet he recalled no lustful intent at that stage, not even any dalliance with fantasy. "I don't think I ever touched them in their private areas," he said, drawing a distinction between those areas and the edges of underwear. "Grabbing them, pulling them, knocking them down. Them jumping on me. It was still just teasing and playing with them. It wasn't like I wanted to have sex with them. Is there a difference?"

• • •

LATELY he'd had fairly open conversations with his family about his crime. Male relatives had talked about their nieces entering adolescence and starting to flirt with them. "And they said, 'Roy, when that happened, we stopped playing with them the same way. We wouldn't let them jump all over us anymore—it scared the daylights out of us. After a certain age, it was no. No to this. No to that. 'Cause things can go a little too far.'"

Listening, I thought of the way Faith's father had spoken to me on the phone one afternoon about his daughter. He was confirming details about what had happened when suddenly he interrupted himself to say how beautiful Faith was, even more gorgeous now than a couple of years ago when Roy had been arrested. "She's killing me," he said. "When I hug her I give her these half-ass hugs." Then, without segue, he volunteered that he never looked at pornographic magazines. "I can appreciate the body, but . . ." His voice trailed off, sounding indifferent. He seemed to want to prove that eros had no hold over him. It was as though the erotic power of his daughter made desire itself uncomfortable, unbearable.

And I thought of my own twelve-year-old daughter, who, along with her younger brother, still loved to be chased through our apartment in a game they called Fee Fi Fo Fum. I, the monstrous giant, chanted the nonsense syllables and twisted her name to fit the rhyme: "I smell the blood of . . ." I dove for her across the couch. She rolled off the cushions and out of reach, shrieking and giggling as she sprinted down the hall from the living room to the master bedroom with me right behind. She darted around the bed. Her body danced on one side while I, on the other, calculated the right moment to lunge. She taunted me, laughing, breathless, telling me I could never catch her, never cook her, never eat her, that this was the night I would starve. And then I made my move. I grabbed her by the wrist, clutched her by the waist. I lifted her into the air and threw her onto the bed. "Now I am cooking you!" I roared. "And then I will devour you!" She cowered in delight.

Constantly Roy tried, but there were so many things he couldn't sort out. How much of the touching had been errant, inadvertent, amid playful mauling? How far beyond the normal had things gone at that stage? Had he gone beyond the normal at all? The questions made him reel; he couldn't settle on single answers. "But was there sexuality behind the games?" he asked himself aloud while we talked—and answered immediately, "Yes."

THE erotic became explicit, he said, when they were in separate rooms, at separate computers. The layout of the house mirrored the one he owned now, many towns away: a series of rooms along a narrow hall, a basement crowded with his guitars and keyboards and recording equipment. His stepdaughter was twelve, though he preferred, when talking to me and perhaps to himself, to say that she was by then fourteen, maybe thirteen. During his introductions in group, he didn't mention how old she was at this point in his story, so for a short while I didn't know her true age. When I read an old article from a local newspaper about the case and told him that it put her age at twelve, he insisted that the article was mistaken. Only after I had asked him a third or fourth time did he call me one morning: he had just phoned his sister and "found out" that the newspaper was right.

When she was twelve, one evening she sent him an instant message. She asked what he was doing. He sat in his office; she was in her bedroom down the hall. He told her he was working on band contracts. She wrote that she was bored, that none of her friends were online. He replied that her brother had been giving their mother trouble, that she was completely different, that she was "a really good little girl."

"She came right back to me and said: 'Roy, you don't know me. I'm not a good girl, I'm a bad girl.'"

He'd always been attracted to the dissolute in the women he dated. He'd been infatuated with the wild streak in Jackie as she had left her husband for him. "I wrote back to her, 'What are you doing?'

"'I'm not going to tell you.'

"It just drew me in. You couldn't have drawn me in any faster. I still remember it. Not excited as in arousal excited, but excited as in I've got to know more. Major adrenaline rush. I felt myself go flush. I felt like I got hot. I told her, 'Gotta get back to work.' She came back on a couple of times with little blurbs like, 'Hurry up and get done, I need somebody to talk to,' and I just ignored those comments because I was already overloaded.

"I finished the contracts I was doing. I got off the computer right after that, and I went immediately downstairs and started playing. That's what I always do when something's really got me; I need to shut it off. I had to shut that off at that moment. I had to calm it down. Put my headphones on. Had my guitar. Sat and played and sang. I have this jazz routine I like doing. I do a jazz version of 'Blue Skies.' 'Polka Dots and Moonbeams'—it's a slow jazz tune. I have a quick fox-trot version of 'I'm in the Mood for Love.' And 'When Sonny Gets Blue'—it's a pretty tune. I have about an hour's worth of music. I just have to concentrate on the chord changes and the progressions, and it clears my mind.

"The only problem is," he almost shouted to me across his kitchen table, "it didn't help."

SOON he loaded his computer with a software program that would allow him to monitor Faith's online conversations. Alone in the house, he stepped back and forth along the hall, between rooms, between computers, making sure his system worked, that she wouldn't be able to detect him reading what she wrote. And the next time she came over and logged on and began chatting with Elizabeth, their words ran across his screen.

"They started talking about school and the boys in school, and Elizabeth said, 'I can't believe you were in the back parking lot with'—I can't remember the kid's name. It was like watching a story. A sexual story, from what Faith started doing, kissing him, to him feeling her, to it just kept progressing. It was like a movie." He followed the progress for weeks, months. He would masturbate after she signed off. "It had your mind so cranked you had to have some relief. I wasn't having sex with my wife. At any point I thought this girl was going to have sex with this boy. That's how intense this was. She told Elizabeth he had her pants off. It really got my motor going. I thought she was going to come on and write that she actually had intercourse with this kid in the back parking lot at school."

He didn't worry that she would walk down the hall and find him reading her words. "Impossible, because my computer didn't face the door, and it would have taken a split second to shut it off. Nobody could catch me, nobody. I'm too good. I'm too good with computers. When I shut the computer off everything was erased. There was no trackable record on those PCs. It was wrong. So wrong. I put myself in such a bad situation, and I just fell into it. I guess that's how a drug addict gets. Once you've fallen into that, it's almost like that's it: now you've got it in your head, and it's not going to go away."

The instant-messaging between him and Faith went on between his monitoring. "She would sign on and see that my computer was online, and she'd say something to me. That's how the conversations started. And I would flip it. She didn't start it sexually. I always flipped it. She didn't do it. She was a kid.

"I said, 'Have you been getting into trouble?' And she said, 'What do you mean by that?'

"'I don't know. You're growing up now. You're starting to turn into a woman.'

"'What do you mean by that?'

"'I don't know.'

"'How are you looking at me?'

"'I'm looking at you as a girl turning into a woman.'

"'What do you mean by that?'

"'You're going to be really attractive when you grow up.'

"'Do you like me that way?'

"'I'm not your father.'"

He suggested that, in front of him, she take off pieces of clothing. She asked what he wanted to see, said no to each request. Online conversation by online conversation, they went back and forth, she asking, he requesting, she saying no, desire surging within him until he suggested that they have sex. She refused.

It was months before her thirteenth birthday when he wrote that he was going to step out of his office and into the kitchen to get a soda. This time, he said that if she wanted to see what he wished to do with her, she should walk into his office and click on a window that would be on his screen. She left her computer and walked to his. When the window opened, a video showed "a man rubbing his penis on a girl's vagina that's been shaved," he told me. A moment later, they passed in the hall. He remembered her calling him "disgusting" and each of them hurrying back to their own PCs. Petrified that she would report him, he begged her over the Internet to meet him on the stairs to the basement music room, promising that he would stay at the bottom. He pleaded his apology as she sat at the top of the stairs. Then she was gone.

AT her father's house, she told her stepmother. Her father was away on a business trip. Her stepmother sent her back to Roy's home so that, assuming he would make his requests yet again, she could print out his words for evidence. The transcript the police read went, in part, like this:

"what do u want again"

"any small thing you want to do"

"like what"

"let me see you"

"what"

"bottom half"

"no. what else"

"in panties"

"y can't you do this stuff with my mom. she's like me and she actually is ur own age"

"i just want to do something with you anything"

He was arrested. In court, he pleaded under the Alford Doctrine, acknowledging that the evidence against him was enough to prove his guilt, and—with decades of probation and the prospect of twenty years in prison if he violated its terms—he had been going to Liddle's sessions now for a year and a half. "I'm so embarrassed," he told me. "I can't believe I did this. I just don't know how I got myself there. I really don't. It makes me sick." And he looked that way—ill, aghast, mortified—whenever he finished his story.

"YOU will see people of varying ages." A woman, one of Liddle's colleagues, stood over Roy, reading from a set of instructions. He sat behind a gray laptop that rested on a metal desk in a small office in the probation building. Her long blond hair fell over a loose sweater. He would be shown one hundred and sixty images on the laptop screen, she informed him. Her voice stayed level, her face expressionless. "Imagine being sexual with the models in the slides."

He wore a black blazer, a tie, sharply pressed khakis. From here he was headed straight to a meeting at work. She told him to score each picture, typing one for "disgusting" up through seven for "highly sexually arousing." He should advance through the images by clicking the return key.

She showed him a practice set: a blond woman in prim white lingerie; a clean-cut man in a plaid shirt and khakis; a boy, who looked to me around twelve, straddling a bicycle with a book bag over his shoulder; a girl around the same age wearing a straw hat and eating strawberries; a pudgy little girl, maybe four, in a blue one-piece swimsuit . . . Liddle's colleague asked Roy if he was ready. Sitting perfectly upright, always demonstrating his obedience, he said that he was. He was left alone with the photographs.

All the men in the circle took the Abel Assessment, an alternative to testing by plethysmograph, at some point during their treatment. It measured erotic preference not by the one-to-seven ratings but by the length of time a man let his eyes linger on each image before clicking to the next. The photos were fairly demure. In the United States, it was illegal for such tests to show pornographic pictures of minors, so to keep things balanced even the adult images held to some degree of decorum. And when, later, I clicked through a set, the distinction between age categories sometimes eluded me. The subjects in the pictures were supposed to represent four plainly separate age groups so categories of attraction could be clearly measured. There were children of two to four, children between eight and ten, adolescents between fourteen and seventeen, and adults at least twenty-two. But some of the eight-to-tens looked to me like young adolescents. And some of the adolescents looked more like youthful adults: they had the kinds of faces and bodies that appeared on billboards selling underwear—an association that turned inward on itself, because those billboard faces and bodies, which defined adult beauty, sometimes belonged to adolescent models.

When Roy finished, he looked shell-shocked, like a patient who'd been through an arduous and shameful diagnostic exam. The information was sent down to the Abel offices in Georgia, and the results were quickly sent up to Liddle. Roy's attractions were for adult females and, slightly more so, for females in the adolescent range.

This put him, Liddle told me, within the realm of ordinary male desire. The preference for adolescents over adults was, he said, a cause for some worry, given Roy's crime. But in itself the strong erotic response to adolescents was entirely normal.

Along the circle sat a few whose Abel scores were plainly aberrant: men drawn above all to preadolescent boys and men drawn powerfully and almost equally to disparate categories, adults and young children, boys and girls. There was a retired accountant who, Liddle said, met the psychiatric definition of a "fixated"—exclusive—pedophile. He had coached sports and built a clubhouse on his property in order to lure the neighborhood boys; he had spanked and groped many over a period of many years, and now, perhaps past the age of desiring anyone—though Liddle suspected otherwise—he lived by himself in a trailer home. On his round mahogany dining table, which was old and scratched, a shiny deck of cards sat on a square of paper towel, as if to keep the cards, at least, unsoiled by all that had long been part of his life.

Most of the group fell somewhere closer to the middle of a continuum: a continuum on which normal occupied a broad and blurry band. And thinking about all the men he'd worked with during the past fourteen years, including the retired accountant, Liddle said, "The difference between me and my guys is a very, very thin line."

Liddle was a marathoner; he'd run Boston in three and a half hours. In his mid-fifties, his deeply sculpted and lined face, and his long, angular body, gave him a look of strength and stoicism. But a muted anxiety lay just beneath his self-restraint, an anxiety not only about the state of his men but about the state of all men, and about himself. It emerged when he spoke about pornography and its proliferation online. Internet porn was "overwhelming, desensitizing." It was "a launching pad for molestation." It was "a nightmare."

"No!" he said, when I asked whether the images might be a way for his men to deal safely with harmful desires: let them masturbate to the pictures and let the longings subside. "That's like an alcoholic saying, 'I'll only have a couple of drinks, I'll only have low-alcohol beer.'" For those in his groups, he felt that even images of adults were dangerous; the legal would only lead to the illicit. But his fear extended beyond his men, beyond what they'd done and might do again with the under-age. Pornography, for him, stood for something ungovernable, something threatening within male desire. He saw the threat everywhere, in movies, in video games, in advertisements. "The meta-message in our society is rape," he said. It was un-clear whether he meant the word to be taken literally or as a suggestion of all that was aggressive, uncontrolled, damaging. "There's so much out there that isn't responsible. I never al-low myself to visit a porn Web site." He'd put a block on his computer to prevent it. He wouldn't let himself so much as fan-tasize about adult strangers. "I have very clear boundaries for myself. If I have deviant thoughts on the train, I think, How comfortable would I be with telling my wife what I'm think-ing? How comfortable would I be with telling my kids? That's how I block myself off." Beyond the bounds of his marriage, all desire was deviant, ominous, liable to lead anywhere.

ONE evening Liddle sent me by e-mail a parable he'd written. It was called "Desire."

There once was a very gifted sculptor who came to a city and was allowed to come in to create his art. He began to work on a beautiful piece of marble he had obtained from a local quarry. While he was carving the stone, a rich patron came by and wanted the piece for his own house. The artist agreed and worked day and night for several weeks to complete the statue for the patron.

Once it was completed, the patron arranged for a large gala for the unveiling of the artwork. He invited the entire town to come to his house. As the moment approached to reveal the statue, there was much anticipation in the minds of the townspeople. The velvet covering was pulled back and there was a gasp of horror from the onlookers.

Each one of the people looking upon the artwork saw something different, something unspeakable. One person saw a man and a child having sexual contact, another saw two men engaged in sex, another saw a woman and an animal in sexual congress, and one saw a man exposing his phallus. Each was sure this was what the piece of art portrayed.

The townspeople reacted by blaming the artist and patron for what they saw. But none of them would talk about what they believed they saw in the marble. They turned on the artist and the patron and forced them to flee the city. Once they were gone, the townspeople destroyed the statue, yet the thoughts and images remained in their hearts.

SOMETIMES when I sat in Roy's kitchen in the evening, with the sky dark outside the windows and the light low over the table and the walls close, I was repelled by his story. I was repelled when I learned about the Internet screen name he'd used—"Freakypeephole"—though he had an explanation: the antidrug anthem he'd written back in the seventies, the song that had brought him his few minutes of airtime, was called "Freaky People." He'd tried for this as his screen name, but it was already taken, and his server had supplied the alternative—he'd accepted Freakypeephole, as a joke, well before his crime. And I was repelled, above all, by his dissembling over Faith's being twelve. The delayed revelation brought home all the more that she had been exactly my daughter's age. The thought of a grown man with my bird-boned, barely pubescent daughter was enough to make my body curl in on itself and enough to make me murderous.

Yet there was excitement in Roy's memories of his aunt. The idea of the slightly older girl beckoning him to the sun room was enviable in itself; that the girl was his mother's sister added a particular electricity. And his stepdaughter's education in the back parking lot; her letting the boy slide her pants over her hips—this was the standard stuff of pornography.

"I was flabbergasted," the owner of the telecommunications repair company said. "I told him, 'Roy, why'd you go off and do something so stupid?'"

I asked the owner about his use of the word "stupid"—it seemed to diminish the crime.

"Listen," he said, "I'm not going to get philosophical, because I'm not smart enough. And I'm not trying to get myself or yourself in trouble. But we're human beings. Everybody has these thoughts. The only thing that separates him from you and me is we didn't act on them."

For the state, Liddle's boss had been watching over and treating men like Roy for twenty years. Before that, he'd been a therapist for child victims of sexual assault. "We want them to be the few, the perverted, the far away," he said about the perpetrators. "We want there to be the clear line. We want there to be the sloped forehead. It just doesn't exist."

A volume of the *Archives of Sexual Behavior*, the world's leading journal of research on sexuality, held an essay by Richard Green, a psychiatrist at the Imperial College School of Medicine in London and a professor emeritus at UCLA. He wrote about a study of around two hundred male university students. "Twenty-one percent reported some sexual attraction to small children. Nine percent described sexual fantasies involving children, five percent admitted to having masturbated to sexual fantasies of children and seven percent indicated they might have sex with a child if not caught." The researchers, Green went on, remarked that "given the probable social undesirability of such admissions, we may hypothesize that the actual rates were even higher." And Green wrote of work done by Kurt Freund: forty-eight Czech soldiers were hooked to a plethysmograph. Viewing a series of slides, "twenty-eight of forty-eight showed penile response to female children age four to ten."

Not many studies had been done, as though to spare everyone the truth. But to think about the Internet or to consider legal history was to deal with something inescapable. Typing in "preteen porn" on AOL's search engine brought a list of sites covering thousands of pages. And until the late nineteenth century in England, the legal age of sexual consent was ten.

"THEY are not monsters. They are us," Joan Tabachnick said. She was the director of public education for Stop It Now!, a national organization devoted to the prevention of child sexual abuse. "It's so much easier to think only of the most sadistic, the most dangerous pedophile. It's very comfortable. It's very uncomfortable to say, 'I know what it means to look at my child as a sexual being—I know what it means to want to touch my child.'"

Words like these made empathy for Roy come all the more readily. And this could lead to minimizing what he had done and attempted to do. But then I would think of the first babysitter who'd taken care of my daughter. I learned about Caroline's past years after she'd left us to become a prison guard. I learned about her past as she told me about her training, about a morning at the Corrections Academy field when she'd clutched her pistol and done what the staff commanded: turned the target's black silhouette into someone she wanted to shoot.

"Are you a pussy or what?" the trainers screamed at classmates around her. "Aim! Shoot the fucking gun! It's your family, he's coming into your house. What you gonna do?" It was pouring. A bank of dark mud rose behind the targets, a place for the bullets to bury themselves. Her new uniform was soaked and clung to her skin. She tried, at first, to control her crying, then realized gratefully that it didn't matter, that no one could tell with the rain. Scarcely an inch taller than five feet, she stood with the target twenty feet away and her instructor spitting, "Who are you home with?"

"It's just me and my kids."

"So what the fuck are you going to do?"

"I'm going to kill him."

I asked whose face and body she had conjured in place of the black silhouette. We sat in her dining room; on the wall above her hung a portrait of a dreadlocked woman. Caroline's own hair surrounded her light brown face in dreadlocks curled so tightly they looked like braided extensions. Her voice was as careful and tight as her hair. She said that she pictured her stepfather.

"No one's known what an encounter was really like. How he would start. What he would do. No one, no one. Because no one really cares to hear. My sister would never; she would die. My mother would probably—no one wants to know that."

Her family was not, she wished to make clear, a chaotic

ghetto stereotype. They had lived in the projects, but her mother had kept their home immaculate and made biscuits and gravy from scratch every weekend. Her stepfather worked steadily and later became a union official. He raised Caroline from the age of one, and throughout her childhood she believed he was her natural father, as he was her younger brothers' and infant sister's. A photograph, taken on a sun-blanched, tree-lined sidewalk when Caroline was around eight, showed him with her and a group of her friends, all gathered close. With a small Afro and fleshy cheeks, he smiles and looks like the kind of man who would lift his eight-year-old stepdaughter onto his shoulders and tour her around their apartment, so she could do what she loved—touch the ceiling and gaze down, from her great height, on the top of the refrigerator.

She was eight when, on her parents' bed, with her mother out on errands and she and her brothers snuggled up to watch television, he started by asking her to scratch his head, to tend his Afro. He asked her to massage his back. In all of this she took pleasure, in the parting and oiling of his hair and the spreading of lotion on his skin, until he told her brothers to leave the room and instructed her to rub his chest. She complied uneasily, moving her hand in tiny circles. "Lower," he said. "Lower, lower, lower."

He led her hand to his penis. Over the next days he forced her mouth. Soon he was turning her facedown on her bed, pulling off her clothes, examining her body silently. He would part her legs; wordlessly he would stroke her back; he would rub himself against her. Whenever she tried to curl or cover herself, he clamped his fingers painfully on her shoulder.

In the sun-blanched photograph, Caroline, wearing a red skirt and black blouse, tugs at a red scarf with both hands, tugs in opposite directions across her throat in symbolic strangling—or mere fidgeting. In another picture, one of the many her stepfather posed and took, she smiles in the park, wearing black patent leather shoes and a white Easter hat, a miniature patent leather pocketbook swinging from her shoulder. Sometimes on Saturday mornings, if her mother went out early to do the laundry, he would wake Caroline, lifting her abruptly out of bed to begin. In one photograph she sleeps beneath a green-and-red striped blanket, head turned to the side and resting on her hand, mouth slack and features serene, hair covered in a pink kerchief.

"I never used to make any sound," she remembered. She stayed quiet through anal rapes that went on, sometimes as frequently as several times in a week, for four years. Trying to soothe at least the physical pain she lived with, she would often spread strips of wet tissue paper between her buttocks as she lay alone in her room. She made sure to wash her blood-stained underwear herself. She would ask her mother not to go to the grocery store or else to let her come along, but she was careful never to beg, for fear that her stepfather would catch on and, as he had once threatened to do, kill her. Then, with the arrival of her first period, she gained what she'd thought of as a grown-up's resolve. Her stepfather had never raped her vaginally; she decided that at least she would try to keep him from ever doing that. And she told herself she was too old now for what he had been doing.

While he listened to jazz one evening in the living room, and while her mother read the Bible in bed and Caroline washed dishes, she planned her words. She went back and forth in her mind about whether to use the word "rape." She walked up and down the hall, from the kitchen to her parents' bedroom door and back again, unable to say anything. At last, she stood beside the bed and told her mother, "Daddy's been having sex with me." When her mother asked if she knew what she was saying, Caroline touched her mouth, then touched her buttocks.

Her stepfather was arrested by housing project police and beaten within her earshot. A prosecutor steered her and her mother away from criminal charges, warning them that it would be her word against his and lamenting the outcome in advance. "I never thought," Caroline told me, "that I'd be— how many years later? I'm almost forty years old—still thinking about this. I never thought it would last this long."

She had three children of her own, a son in college and two younger twin daughters in a junior high school program for the gifted. As for herself, she said, "Just take something with very intricate parts and just shake the whole thing up and flip it upside down and stand it up. I mean, you're not going to have a clue." She talked about sometimes still missing her stepfather, about feeling somehow rejected by him, and she described a life so permeated by a sense of her own strangeness that, despite the success of her kids, she felt utterly uncertain of her judgments about everything. "All the norms that you're taught are taken away from you," she explained the effect of those four years. "It makes everything foreign."

Throughout those years, her stepfather had licked her vagina, the sensations pleasurable beneath her fear and revulsion. And the legacy of her childhood had led to adult lovemaking during which she imagined having vaginal intercourse with him. She would picture herself with him, but as she was now: "an older woman, experienced, like I was giving him something." It was the only way she could reach orgasm.

• • •

DOWN the hall from Meredith Chivers, the psychologist at the edge of the forest of female sexuality, Ray Blanchard and James Cantor believed that the pictures of the brain they had recently taken and studied all but proved nature's dominance over nurture, biology's primacy over experience, in setting the direction of desire. The research appeared almost unprecedented. (One precursor was a controversial study published by the sexologist Simon LeVay in 1991: autopsies of gay and straight men detected a difference, corresponding to sexual orientation, in the size of a minuscule cluster of cells in the hypothalamus.) Blanchard and Cantor radiated triumph. Blanchard was a compact man with a disciplined gray beard; there was efficiency in the way he looked, and, in the way he spoke, dismissiveness when he mentioned those who opposed him.

"In graduate school I started in clinical psych," he said, "and it was a hardcore behavioral therapy department. You were taught to apply methods, learned in the laboratory with rats and pigeons, to humans." Behavioral conditioning was the prevailing theory of his professors, and he had rebelled. "The emperor has no clothes," he recalled sensing. He couldn't pinpoint the reasons for his early skepticism. He seemed almost to ascribe his judgment to his own superior instinct, to biology.

He switched, in school, from the clinical department to the experimental, from a focus on humans to lab work with animals. "And what I discovered was that the animal experts weren't talking so much about learned behavior anymore. Instinctive behavior, prepared behavior—these were becoming the things. So you had clinicians teaching that you can just apply these learning principles established beyond doubt in the animal laboratory, while the people doing animal research were saying, 'Well, it's not really like that.'" Ever since, Blanchard's career had followed—and, in a small way, forged—the path of scientific culture toward medical, physiological explanations for human behavior. And now, in the infinitely complex realm of eros, he felt that he and Cantor held confirmation.

In the lab at one end of their floor, a technician had hooked a plethysmograph to the one hundred and twenty-seven men who were Blanchard and Cantor's current subjects, and he had tested for arousal to the young. "I've studied mind, body, and soul," the technician told me; he had earned master's degrees in psychology, medical science, and religion. "And here I am measuring dicks." He had seen, he guessed, thirty-two hundred, and he often conducted an informal interview before strapping on the glass tube and securing the wires and leaving the subject alone, pants around ankles, with the slide show. For his own curiosity, he liked to ask, "If I had a video clip of your mind in the last ten seconds before you climax during sex, what would I see?" He marveled at how few men, including those who were excited most by adult women, said that the ten-second video would be filled with the women they were with.

The current subjects were split nearly equally between pedophiles and what Blanchard called "teleophiles"—"the normal guys," he translated, though with a hint of irony: a recent study of his own jibed with those Richard Green had cited. Normal didn't mean uninterested in the young. Measured by plethysmograph, teleophilic heterosexuals were aroused most by pictures of female adults, but significantly, too, by female pubescents and, less so but still markedly, by female children. There was no mistaking ordinary men's erotic response to very young girls when their reaction to female children was compared to their negligible responses to slides of males of any age, or when it was compared to their indifference to a neutral picture: a photograph of a pond surrounded by the bare limbs of trees in winter. Teleiophilic homosexuals adhered to their own analogous continuum. And the pattern held in reverse for the pedophilic.

After their sessions with the plethysmograph, the hundred and twenty-seven men had slid into the cylinder of an MRI machine, and images had been taken of their brains.

A magenta cat floated on the computer screen, body tilted upright, belly exposed, eyes bulging. Its limbs were grotesquely short, except for one long foreleg that swiped at the air. An amorphous teal creature sat behind the cat, tending like a servant to the floating animal's back, stroking. Below the cat stood a pair of slender beings: twins, one magenta and one teal, as though the cat and its servant were lovers and these were their children. Little teal amoebas were suspended all around them.

The colored shapes were superimposed on a white-and-gray side view of the human brain. The cat and the servant, the twins and the amoebas were areas where a difference existed between pedophilic and teleiophilic brains, with the magenta forms signifying differences in the right hemisphere and the teal indicating distinctions in the left. The MRI pictures of the two groups of brains had been analyzed and compared, minuscule point by minuscule point, for quantity of white matter. Within the magenta and teal areas, Cantor, an elfin man in a black sweater vest, explained, "the more pedophilic a person is, the more the amount of white matter goes down."

Specialized technicians—"my two imaging geeks," Cantor

adoringly called the young man and woman who spent their days rotating, slicing, and tinting images as they rendered representations of the brain on their computers—had transformed the quantitative analysis into graphics that made visual sense of the comparisons. And it seemed right that the outcome would look like a surrealist's vision. The surrealists had given shape to the subconscious, to anarchic and bewildering desires that could be buried but never killed off. Here, on the screen, was the science of lust turned into art.

And here was proof, it seemed, that a divergence of desire was rooted in the anatomy of the brain, proof that pointed to the prenatal in molding sexuality. Blanchard and Cantor acknowledged that the physiological differences could somehow be caused by pedophilic experience; they foresaw that those who refused to accept the determinative power of biology would insist on making this argument as soon as the study was published. But the argument, they felt, would be strained, especially given an earlier discovery they'd made—that pedophilic men are about three times more likely than teleiophiles to be left-handed. The statistical link was glaring, and handedness is set prenatally. Now, with their current results, it seemed logically undeniable that pedophilia, or at least a strong predisposition toward pedophilia, was determined prenatally, too.

Even about the evidence that perhaps one-third of sexual abusers had, as children, been abused themselves, Blanchard and Cantor were dismissive. The data were overly reliant on self-reported, unverified histories, Cantor argued. And Chivers's husband, the researcher Michael Seto, who supported Blanchard and Cantor's conclusions, said that while he did credit the link between being abused and abusing, this didn't contradict the idea of pedophilia's prenatal origin. The abused might have a related inborn trait that made them psychologically vulnerable to, or more likely to receive, adult advances, he suggested. Or being abused might be "a trigger" that, later, set off the prenatally loaded tendency.

"Terror," Cantor said, remembering his feelings as the early results of the brain imaging had come in, and had seemed, for a short while, inconclusive. "My heart was beating fast. I thought, I'll never find anything. There's nothing here."

"Thank God!" Blanchard recalled his reaction as the patterns of difference in the temporal and parietal lobes had become more and more clear with the help of the imaging geeks.

And now, showing me and Michael Seto the latest computer-generated graphics of differentiation, Cantor was thrilled. His snug sweater vest seemed unable to contain the exuberance within him. "Isn't that the hottest thing in the world?" he asked. He directed one of the technicians to click slowly through a series: the differences viewed from dozens of vantage points and highlighted in red and yellow and green. "It doesn't get any cooler than that!" he exclaimed. Then he told the man to rotate one of the graphics; he wanted us to admire it from all angles. With the technician manipulating the computer's mouse, a large, three-dimensional, liver-shaped glob flew toward us, paused, spun slowly, paused again, and seemed to pose in front of us like a runway model, challenging anyone to gaze her way and doubt the supremacy of what she had to offer. "The proof is staring us in the face!" Cantor declared.

Posters of three Michelangelo sibyls, the Delphic, Libyan, and Eritrean seers, hung above Cantor's desk. "I just want to know how the sexual brain works," he said. "What makes the human brain tick when it comes to sexuality. That's our thing. Etiology." He made it clear that he was less driven by the wish to have some practical effect in the field of child sexual abuse than by the wish to know how we become who we are in the world of eros.

With the aid of magnetic resonance imaging, with the assistance of his geeks, with the power of equipment and techniques that hadn't yet been invented, Cantor wanted to become a kind of seer. But, exultant though he was over the revelations in magenta and teal, he knew he hadn't yet seen with enough precision, not at all. The vast differences between the pedophilic and teleiophilic brains, as detected by the MRI machine, were almost certainly too generalized, too vague. The magenta and teal reflected not only the divergent directions of lust but also the fact that pedophilic brains held any number of associated conditions, "a constellation of symptoms" having little or nothing to do with sex, Cantor suspected. As his and Blanchard's thinking went, something had happened in the womb, a "perturbation," as they called it, probably a chemical event, a toxin introduced by anything from maternal drug use to infection to some agent in the environment, the introduction coinciding with a particular developmental period for the fetus. The result was an array of abnormalities in the white matter. Somewhere within the magenta and teal was the exact area of distinction that led to pedophilia, but so far Cantor and Blanchard had no method to eliminate the irrelevant regions. "We haven't hit *it* yet," Cantor said, and he guessed that the precise point of relevance might be too tiny for present technology to pick up. "A three-dimensional pixel is called a voxel. A voxel is about one millimeter cubed. But of course a fiber in the brain is much smaller than that. So if there are fine differences they may be too thin for an MRI ever to be able to see."

Our conversation drifted to the men whose brains he studied. About those who preferred children, he said, "I don't think any of them are quite happy. I don't think I would be quite happy if I realized that I would never be permitted the sexual partners I find most attractive: that's it; there's nothing I can do about it. It's easy to understand why a lot of them ask for sex drive—reducing medications. They don't want a sex drive they have to spend the rest of their lives resisting, that they're never allowed to express. It's easier to try to live without the sex drive altogether."

He spoke about the near-absence of sexual aberration among animals. In humans, "higher parts of the brain have taken over things done by lower parts in other species. And it appears that one of those things is sexual behavior." The result, he said, was not a complexity worth celebrating. "More things can go wrong. It's like with each new version of Windows we just end up with more problems."

And the problems are compounded by constancy. Most animals have their mating seasons; humans are prepared for sex year-round, and so continually prone to torment.

Was there, I asked, any chance that someone with a dominant desire for children could move to a different point on the continuum, any hope that he could subordinate that lust to another; was there any possibility for real change?

Beneath the three sibyls Cantor's voice flattened. It lost the buoyancy that came with his talk about the science of eros; he was no longer peering into unknowns nor thrilled by his discoveries.

"Not that I'm aware of," he said. Biology was the beginning, and biology was the end.

"MASTURBATORY reconditioning," Blanchard wrote later in an e-mail, answering a question I'd sent about the brain's capacity for reconfiguration, a capacity known as neuroplasticity. If stroke victims could, through relentless and painstaking practice, stir their brains to sprout new neural wiring that allowed them to walk, to speak, might the physiology of the brain, I wondered, be similarly plastic when it came to desire? "I don't recall exactly when the notion of masturbatory reconditioning was introduced," he wrote. "Probably back in the 1960s, when a number of behavior therapy procedures, based on conditioning experiments with rats, dogs, and pigeons, were first applied to human patients. The basic procedure was that a patient with pedophilia, fetishism, or (in those days) homosexuality would be instructed to masturbate, with a *Playboy* magazine within easy reach. When the patient started to approach orgasm, he was supposed to grab the magazine and focus intently on the nude adult female just before and during ejaculation. This was supposed to establish erotic interest in adult females.

"One would expect that such a procedure, if effective, would have swept the world. I think that would have been true even if it turned masturbation into a tiresome obligation. In fact, the treatment has been quietly abandoned, like many of the animal lab–based therapy inventions of the 1960s (although one can, of course, find pockets here and there where these procedures are still recommended)."

CANTOR talked about the course his career had taken the way Blanchard did, as beyond his control. To ask why he'd become a sexologist, or why, as a sexologist, he'd been drawn to prove physiological explanations for attraction, was "like asking a twig how did it float down the river," he said. "I'm a twig, I'm in the water, and this is where I ended up."

It was different two hundred miles to the northeast, in Ottawa, where Paul Fedoroff—like Berlin and Blanchard, one of the world's best-known sexologists—spoke about how he'd come to treat a legion of paraphiliacs, among them a man who had sex with horses, a woman who had stroked herself so frequently her vagina was covered in sores, and an array of pedophiles, all of whom, Fedoroff believed, could change. During medical school, he said, he'd met a psychologist, a researcher whose focus was sexuality. "He told me about the case of an NFL football player who'd been arrested for exhibitionism. The man was a quarterback, a star. He'd married a Miss America or someone like that. And this psychiatrist said, 'Think about it. Here's a guy who's the envy of every man in the States. He's the quarterback of a winning football team. Every weekend literally millions of people watch everything he does. He's married to the prettiest woman of the year in the U.S. And even with all that, for some reason he goes out and exposes himself.' The league had known about the problem and covered it up for some time, but this apparently was one time too many. He lost his job, his huge salary, his wife. And this psychologist said, 'There's something interesting here.'"

Fedoroff had padded cheeks and a sharp nose, a soft middle amid a stretch of height. There was a mix of softness and superiority in his face and body. And then there was the sheer enthusiasm of his clothes. His suits flaunted the thick pinstripes of the moment; they were so current in their style, he looked almost like a dandy. A rim of gray hair, some of it tossed untidily over the top of his head, undercut the dandyism. But the enthusiasm, the energy—he saw patients and met with colleagues and addressed seminars from early morning till after dark without even a break for coffee—were unmitigated.

"I've fooled around with dogs," a patient told him one afternoon, his eyes shut tight, as though against the truths he was confiding. "Not mounting—masturbating. I have relationships with horses. I don't know if I want to stop. If given the choice, I'd choose a horse over a woman."

"Why?" Fedoroff asked quietly. He leaned back in his leather desk chair, a bright tie bringing extra flourish to the high fashion of his suit, while across from him, on the couch, the man sat upright in a dingy T-shirt and dusty khakis. He was portly, with a light brown mustache.

"The trust factor," he said. He added that he had a girlfriend.

"Isn't that preferable?"

"I find I'm closer to horses."

Fedoroff's office was in a small, square hospital building with low ceilings and floors of bleary linoleum. Above Fedoroff's head hung a print by Chagall: a floating couple engaged in an airborne kiss. The scene looked, at first, blissful, banal; the woman clutched a bouquet of flowers while her lips met her lover's. Yet on second glance, all was askew.

The patient acknowledged that there might be emotional limitations in his relationships with horses. He explained that he'd had some run-ins within the zoophile community over this very point. "They say there's a husband and wife bond between the human and the animal." His feelings didn't go quite that far. Still, he kept returning to the trust factor. "You're not going to have an animal try to hurt you emotionally. You're not going to have an animal make fun of you." He didn't think he'd always been attracted this way. He believed it was a product of human betrayal.

When he touched himself, he did so with horses in mind. Whenever he could, he made love to one of the mares at a local stable. He'd come to Fedoroff's office out of fear: he didn't want to change, but he didn't want to get caught; sex with horses could be punished with years in prison. His dream was of a life across the border and down in Missouri and back in the past. "Missouri," he said, "was once a legal state."

He saw his lovemaking as part of natural progression. "People have been training horses for thousands of years. Long ago horses didn't have people on their backs. They didn't have bits in their mouths. Now they do." He was merely taking the next step. And he was careful to do no harm, to take no advantage, never to mount the young. "They don't really know what sex is. Their drive isn't there. It's like a child—they don't really know what's going on." Nor would he persist with an unwilling adult. He could tell when desire was returned. "Mares are very vocal."

Fedoroff took all this in without reaction except, once, to straighten his tie and, now and then, to suggest gently that change was possible. The patient stayed focused on immediate fears: arrest, disease. He asked Fedoroff if illness was communicable between animals and humans, and in reply the psychiatrist asked if he used condoms.

"Me and my human partner use protection. Me and my equine partners don't."

Fedoroff scheduled another appointment for him several weeks away. He tended to see his patients individually every month or so, though many came weekly to group sessions. He monitored them and often medicated them and checked up on the therapy some of them received elsewhere. The zoophile didn't yet want treatment of any kind. "If he agreed," Fedoroff told me after the man left, "I would try to steer him more strongly toward humans." Then he went out into the waiting area to greet his next patient.

Lust, Fedoroff believed, was analogous to language. "People are born without language," he said, "but with a genetic makeup that allows them to acquire and express any of the languages that exist in the world. And the language they end up speaking is determined by who they're raised by. At about the age of two their mother tongue is set, so that even though a person can learn new languages the fact is that there's a basic hardwired one. Even with people who are multilingual, if you ask what their mother tongue is, they can tell you. And if they can't, if they say 'I speak these languages equally well,' and you ask, 'When you calculate numbers in your head what language do you use?' there will be one answer." It was similar with sexuality. Infinite possibilities narrowed early on; what John Money, Berlin's mentor, had called "the lovemap" took shape. But all was not over; the lovemap was not unmalleable. "If you buy that it is," he went on, "then you tend to think like neurologists do: diagnose and *adios*. It's a fatalistic approach, and over the years I've discovered that it's not right. Because of course people are capable of learning and developing second languages. I'm not sure that you can get rid of the original interest. But you can become less dependent on it by developing new desire."

Fedoroff assumed that desire was shaped by all sorts of factors, biological and experiential, weighted differently in different people. Unlike Blanchard and Cantor, he wasn't bent on proving nature's predominance over nurture, though he was fascinated by the evolutionary, the biological. Thinking about why certain body parts and objects were frequent targets of paraphilic desire, he said, "People have asked exactly the same question about why there are certain things we are more likely to be phobic about. Heights, the dark, wiggly objects—these are phobogenic across cultures. One answer is that people have been naturally selected for these fears. People with fear of heights are probably more likely to have children than people who don't. So using the analogy with fetishes, there are things we're genetically predisposed to sexualize. Characteristic odors. You can look at animals and see the power of odors in reproductive behavior. It's not too much of a leap to say that humans have odor-driven sexual pathways, and that many of the things that are fetishized have or are associated with musky smells—feet, shoes, undergarments." Fetishes, like phobias, were a legacy of evolutionary advantage, an expression of desired traits taken to excess or diverted to related targets.

Sometimes Fedoroff's mind seemed close to exploding with theories. "I resist single answers because they all turn out to be wrong." His etiological explanations included the role of shame and fear in spurring orgasm. Some paraphiliacs, he thought, suffered from a "sticky switch" governing their parasympathetic and sympathetic nervous systems, two branches of the autonomic circuitry that regulates heart rate, sweating, breathing, salivation. The parasympathetic system controls arousal while the sympathetic sends us into the ecstasy of orgasm. "The natural progression during sex is that the parasympathetics are set off, and at some point when we become sufficiently aroused a switch flips and the sympathetics kick in and we start to have an orgasm. But the poor paraphiliac has a sticky, sluggish switch and needs to do something extreme to get the sympathetics going." Besides orgasm, the sympathetic system takes control in situations of emergency, and Fedoroff's theory was that some paraphiliacs use the deviant or forbidden to stoke their sense of mortification or danger—to create the emotional emergency that would open up the sympathetic pathways and drive things on toward climax.

He mentioned a patient, a heterosexual woman, who sought treatment because she'd lost the ability to climax with her regular partner. Sex with a succession of men in the same evening; videos of women copulating with animals; making videos of herself masturbating—these sent her toward orgasm. Satisfying sex with her partner seemed a hopeless cause "until," Fedoroff wrote in a journal article, "it was discovered that she consumed large amounts of L-tryptophan, available in health food stores, to help her sleep. This substance is metabolized into serotonin, which is known to cause difficulty reaching orgasm. She was advised to discontinue taking L-tryptophan. Soon afterward, her ability to reach orgasm through intercourse with her partner returned, and with it, her paraphilic interest in group sex, exhibitionism, and zoophilia disappeared."

After the man who mounted horses, Fedoroff's next patient was a girl who looked to be in her late teens. Her blue hair formed a spiky plumage above her pale, round face. She wore heavy black boots and a beige fleece with a stitched outline of a lion's head decorating the front. The stitching wasn't prominent; the lion's face and mane were ethereal, like the specter of something aggressive or untamable that lived within her. Once, she'd masturbated compulsively, abrading herself until her genitals were disfigured by sores. She'd humped herself with broom handles. She'd fondled dogs. She'd been living in a group home; her groaning during masturbation had unsettled the staff, and there had been accusations that she molested younger residents. Now, under Fedoroff's care, an anti-androgen curtailed her erotic drives. But he didn't think her problems were permanent. He didn't think the chemical restraint would always be needed. He suspected that she had an obscure genetic disorder, that her particular array of symptoms pointed to a certain missing chromosome, yet as he leaned toward her, from his chair toward the couch, he drew her a comforting graph with a line that zigged and zagged but climbed ever upward, the zags representing setbacks but the climb representing inevitable overall improvement. "I know you want to live a normal life," he said. "There are going to be some bumps along the way. But I think you will." It wasn't clear exactly how normality would be accomplished and maintained as the drugs were removed, but the girl listened, unquestioning, looking at least a little reassured.

Her case reminded him of another, and after he'd led her out with a few more soft, upbeat words, he described a patient with an even more rare genetic disorder, Lesch-Nyhan syndrome. The young man had to live strapped down to a chair; unrestrained, he would gnaw off his own fingers and tear off his penis. The compulsion to mutilate and get rid of his own extremities was caused by a deficient supply of a single enzyme. "It's amazing that it's just one enzyme that keeps us from doing these things," he said. Another symptom, for his patient, was that change—any change—was excruciating, unbearable. But the man's parents, whom he lived with, had learned to adapt. Every night they moved pieces of furniture, so that change was the soothing constant. And understanding that their son needed some sort of sex life, they designed a special apparatus that allowed him to masturbate without granting him the freedom to dismember himself.

Fedoroff adored the ingenuity of the parents; it fed his faith in solutions. His trust in the possibility of setting things right dated back to a truck driver transvestite decades ago. At the time, Fedoroff had been a psychiatric resident going through a required period of psychoanalytic training, but when more than a year of talking brought no change in the cross-dressing, a mentor suggested that he shift his focus from treating the paraphilia to addressing the patient's anxiety. Fedoroff decided to try a new medication, buspirone.

"Soon I get a call from the guy's wife. I've never heard from this woman before. She said, 'What is that medicine you put my husband on?' I said, 'Well, it's this new antianxiety drug; is he less anxious?' And she said, 'No, he's as anxious as he ever was, but don't ever take him off it.' 'Why's that?' And she said, 'Because we're having the best sex we've ever had in our lives.'

"So I had the truck driver come in. This was a macho guy, but during sex he'd had to have lingerie on, or have intense fantasies about wearing it. And his wife had picked up on the fantasies; she described it as his being completely tuned out. And now he said, 'I don't know why, but I don't have to do that anymore. I can have sex with my wife, and I don't have to think about lingerie at all. This has never happened to me in my life.'

"We took him off the medication, and six weeks later he couldn't function unless he was thinking about lingerie. Put him back on and the problem disappeared again. But a long while later I called him and asked, 'Are you still taking it?' He told me no. He kept a bottle of it in the cupboard, just in case. But he didn't need it. I'm quite convinced there had been a fundamental change in his lovemap."

Fedoroff's theory was that the buspirone had eased the "sticky switch" that engaged the sympathetic nervous system during sex. With the switch working smoothly, making ordinary love with his wife became a thorough pleasure. He'd been able to develop a second language, to become fully functional within it, and eventually the drug was no longer necessary.

Pedophiles, too, might learn to manage without their mother tongue. Fedoroff talked about putting them through a second puberty. His plan depended on the idea that everyone had once been pedophilic. As children we'd had our primary crushes on other children. For most of us, our preferred objects of desire grow older as we do, at least through puberty and for several years beyond. But for the pedophile, Fedoroff thought, something had gone awry around puberty's onset—and the solution was to set the patient back into a prepubertal state. This could be accomplished, at least as far as the sex drive went, by giving anti-androgens. With the lust for children out of the way, emotionally romantic attachments with adults would be given a second chance to develop. Then the dosage of anti-androgen could be gradually reduced, allowing sexuality to join up with the romantic sentiments.

It was a theory somewhat like the one Berlin had described as central to Money's thinking—and as disproved. What made Fedoroff confident that an attraction to adults would gradually rival the longing for children wasn't fully apparent. He hadn't yet tested his idea, though he intended to soon. His self-assurance seemed to rely on another analogy: on thinking not only in terms of language but in terms of cuisine. "I tell my guys, 'What you've been doing is like eating at fast food restaurants. Your fast food days are over. The gourmet dining experience is coming. If all you've experienced is sex with children, you have no idea what it's like to have sex with someone who can actually reciprocate and play on the same level as you. Once you've had that, once you've had gourmet food, you won't want to go back.'"

The metaphors seemed to buoy him above all doubt. And to be around him was to float above darkness and to feel that desire need hold no threat, no anguish. "If you haven't noticed," he declared one evening at a dinner party at his home, "I'm very sex-positive." The house embodied a mix of the intellectual and the sensual. A sculpted relief of three nude backsides decorated one bathroom. A large library, lined with built-in bookcases that rose from floor to ceiling, opened onto a small indoor swimming pool. On the floor above, a balcony in the living area overlooked the water and whoever might be swimming or floating languidly. Directly behind the house, which was a ten-minute drive from downtown, a tributary to the Rideau Canal ran past. Fedoroff could fish for carp from his back deck. And the force of this water, seen through the windows, seemed to stitch the bookish and erotic elements of the house inextricably together.

At the opposite end of the dining table from where he sat, Fedoroff's wife, who had served takeout Indian food for the occasion, joked about her cooking with one of his interns. "He has to put up with my experimenting."

Overhearing, he called across the table, "Are you talking about our sex life?"

Someone asked whether his patients ever turned in any strange sex toys, whether he kept a collection.

"I'm his sex toy," his wife yelled out.

She had a tousle of long hair, dyed blond with dramatic dark roots. She wore black pants that clung to her slender hips and a tank top that showed off her arms, her breasts. They'd met when she was a psychiatric nurse on a ward where he was doing rounds. To their guests, she told a story about being trained to wrestle unruly patients to the ground. She told stories, too, about a pornography convention she and Fedoroff had attended because of some research he'd done. She'd had her picture taken perched on Larry Flynt's lap, in his wheelchair. And Nina Hartley, a porn star "known for her ass," she said, had patted her on the butt, which she had taken, she recounted, smiling half-ironically, as a particular tribute.

Considering the perfect body and profligate hair and brazen conversation of his wife, I thought, No wonder he has such an optimistic vision of the erotic. Everything is easy—reality is fantasy—in his house. Then, amid the laughter that followed the Nina Hartley story, his wife said, "I used to be insecure about my boobs," and explained raucously that they had been much smaller before she'd contracted breast cancer and gone for prosthetics. The laughter doubled, hers the loudest of all. So they'd had their share of darkness, I thought. There had been anguish to fight through.

FEDOROFF didn't deny that his metaphoric reasoning was imperfect, that his own analogies could work against him. A person might gain fluency in a second language, and might live for years far from his native soil, but still have a longing to return home and speak his mother tongue. A person might discover haute cuisine, develop his palate, and take keen pleasure in the food's complexity, but still have a hankering for McDonald's. Yet Fedoroff believed that stubborn desires could be dealt with in the pedophile—partly through pornography. He and Patrick Liddle thought in opposite ways. Liddle wanted his men nowhere near pornography, not even images of adults; he wanted lust circumscribed, narrowed, in some ways negated, for fear that it could lead so easily to the uncontrollable. For Fedoroff, desire wasn't pervaded by threat. He ran groups like Liddle's, gathered molesters around him in circles of chairs, gave them a place to gain self-control. Yet he didn't seem anxious that they might be one step away from molesting again. At the dinner party, he said that staring at child pornography could help the men; they could masturbate, diminishing their urges, their yearning to speak the mother tongue, their wish for fast food. He mentioned a study showing that during a period when the availability of child pornography had increased in Denmark, sexual offenses against children had declined. The same had been shown in Japan. Fedoroff encouraged his molesters to fantasize. Fantasy hurt no one. Touching yourself hurt no one. And with the craving sated, the patient could turn his attention back to developing the second language, the taste for the gourmet.

One evening, as Fedoroff led a group that held a range of offenders—against children, against adults, against animals—a patient who'd assaulted a woman confided that he'd been looking at pornography online. A Muslim in the circle, another patient, inveighed against this: "Our scholars tell us that looking leads to touching and this will destroy." He had a thick black beard and wore white leather Converse high-tops. He could have been speaking for Liddle. And Fedoroff replied, "Billions of people find pornography pleasurable. It's okay. There's nothing in the Koran about *Playboy*. There's nothing in the Koran about X-rated videos."

"Not specifically." The Muslim stared Fedoroff down.

But nothing could shake him. One morning, a patient settled himself on Fedoroff's couch for one of his periodic check-ins. With neatly cropped dark hair and a blue crewneck sweater, the man talked about having just found a girlfriend online, using the dating service Lavalife.

"Do you have a profile?" Fedoroff asked blandly.

"Uh-huh."

"What do you say about yourself?"

"Just a paragraph."

"Now, you have some special sexual interests—do you mention any of those?"

"Nah."

The special sexual interests included binding women in a certain position, arms behind their torsos, accentuating their breasts. Twice the man had kidnapped women from parking lots, driven them out into the country, forced them from the car, used large screw clamps to bind their ankles and arms and a knife to slice off outer clothing. During one of these assaults, the sight of the woman in his favorite position had been enough to make him come without any touching. The other time, he'd been about to rape his victim, threatening her with an ice pick, but stopped when she begged him not to go on. He'd spent a few years in prison. A few months ago he'd been arrested for soliciting a prostitute. As he talked with his patient, Fedoroff turned to me and explained that in Ottawa prostitution was legal but soliciting a prostitute was not. The irony amused him. He seemed concerned by the societal schizophrenia reflected in the policy. He didn't seem worried by the fact that his patient had been negotiating to bind the prostitute in his preferred way. He didn't seem too concerned that the man was free and courting women on Lavalife. He didn't seem panicked that the man's dose of medication was apparently not enough to subdue a desire that, the patient told him, sometimes felt "like anticipating a fix of heroin." Fedoroff told me later that trying to arrange for a prostitute to be tied up was a sign of significant progress—a move away from the violently coercive and toward the consensual. He didn't see it as a sign that the man might soon again be wielding an ice pick.

The patient went on his way, out Fedoroff's door and out into the world. The psychiatrist mentioned to me that successful phallometric testing for tendencies toward violent, coercive sex was difficult. Among all men, sexually violent pictures and audiotapes were "too generally arousing."

At the dinner party, he mused about giving sex offenders Viagra. A parallel approach had worked with AIDS patients. "People say, 'Men with AIDS on Viagra?' They're incredulous. But men with AIDS get erection problems, especially when they're put on all these drugs. They stop using condoms. Instead, you prescribe Viagra so they'll have safe sex."

For offenders who had trouble getting erect "in appropriate contexts," he went on, Viagra might help in learning second languages. He imagined writing prescriptions for pedophiles. Then came another metaphor to go with language and cuisine: his plan to interrupt the sex drive with anti-androgens was "like an orthopedic surgeon breaking an arm intentionally in order to let it mend and redevelop into a healthy limb."

The metaphors were seductive, each one seeming beyond argument, each one substantiating the others. Couldn't we indeed learn fluency in second languages? Wasn't a four-star meal more compelling than a Big Mac? Didn't orthopedic surgeons sometimes do exactly as Fedoroff said in treating a malformed arm or leg? Fedoroff seemed a visionary. "Some guys spend their time in the lab," he said over dessert. "They're the ones who win the Nobel. But—all right, I'm drunk—I want to change the world. I might not succeed. But that's what I want."

He longed to prove that desire could take fundamentally new paths. To succeed with pedophiles would draw everyone's attention. The prevailing opinion was Cantor's, that transformation for such men was impossible: talk therapy couldn't accomplish it, conditioning couldn't accomplish it. The only hopes were to extinguish eros with drugs or to teach techniques of self-restraint, the way Liddle did, and pray that they were enough.

You *are* drunk, I said silently to Fedoroff at dinner, but then thought of a tribe ten thousand miles away in the jungle highlands of Papua New Guinea. An anthropologist, Gilbert Herdt, had lived among them during the 1970s and discovered that the erotic lives of their boys and men passed through stages as transformative as any redirection that Fedoroff envisioned.

The Sambia, Herdt had called the tribe in reporting what he'd found, using a pseudonym to protect the people from an onslaught of Western attention.

Sambian boys, at around the age of seven, began performing fellatio on the teenage males of their clans. The act was considered necessary to fill the young boys with semen. The fluid would then manufacture more of itself inside the boys' bodies, but to build up a sufficient base in order to create a life's supply, the boys had to give frequent blow jobs. In this way, both the young, who swallowed, and the teens, who climaxed, were performing a service for the survival of their people. As the teenagers grew into men, they passed beyond homosexuality, took wives, and impregnated their women. But in addition to allowing for reproduction, the homosexual rites offered pleasure, not only for the teenagers but, Herdt observed, for the boys, who had their favorite partners. Sambian males seemed to pass seamlessly from being homosexual givers of oral sex to being homosexual receivers of oral sex to being heterosexual.

Audibly, loudly, despite the vast distance and the decades that had passed, Herdt's research argued that the direction of lust could change—easily. It could change according to a culturally constructed system; the learned seemed far more potent than the congenital, the prenatal. And I'd sensed this often as I spent time with the paraphilic.

One night, on my way to a lecture the Baroness was giving to a society of sadists and masochists, I glanced up through my taxi window at a billboard in Times Square. The model's face filled me with a wanting so keen I felt bereft. Then I walked down a set of gray metal stairs and entered the fluorescently lit basement room where the Baroness was speaking. The dominatrixes in the audience had bodies ranging from the thick to the obese; their faces were plain. Yet the room was charged with the craving, the devotion, the love of the submissives who surrounded them. Three hours later, as I headed back through Times Square in another taxi, the woman on the billboard was almost unrecognizable. Her looks had little effect on me. I hadn't adopted the ways of seeing that suffused the basement air, but I had absorbed them. I hadn't become enamored of the obese and plain, but my way of seeing had shifted. It would shift back. It wouldn't take long. A rush of conventional culture, beamed through the taxi windows from the rest of the neighborhood's huge and luminous advertisements, would be enough to carry out the reversion.

IF Sambian males could change so radically, couldn't Michael Thayer? With tight blond curls and a way of locking his gaze to the eyes of anyone he spoke to, he attended one of Fedoroff's groups each week. He had licked and sucked his young daughter's genitals, and been sentenced to treatment. Fedoroff had put him on a strong dose of Lupron. Before that, merely reading a book with a child character could overwhelm him. He talked about finishing a novel in which a boy was killed. "I was grieving over this child. Responding as though I was in love. And it was like that in my life. For the conversation, for the teaching, for the sexual—the same as you'd fall for an adult, I would fall for a child."

The Lupron put him "totally to sleep." He lost not only all interest in sex but almost all inclination to socialize. He worked as a groundskeeper outside a government complex, weeding flower beds, scouring graffiti. "People were always around me, asking me for directions. This included children," he recalled in an e-mail he sent me. "I was a little nervous being around the kids, but that is all. Everything was fine with my attractions."

Then, abruptly, though there had been no change in dosage, he "woke up." It was Canada Day, and the grounds were thronged. "It seemed that every child in the city was there playing and running around. I had to walk through groups of them to get to the various work sites. It was okay for the first couple of hours, but eventually my defenses and nerves broke down. The thoughts were so severe that I had to rush home. I spent the next two days alone in my apartment virtually in tears. The thoughts lasted for two weeks and refused to give up. It was so bad that I almost approached my probation officer to ask her to call the police and take me into custody."

But something still more strange came next. By the third week, he said, the torturous longing for children faded, and by the fourth it disappeared, replaced by interest in adult women. The substitution was far more swift than anything Fedoroff had imagined. Michael remembered that when he told Fedoroff what had happened, the psychiatrist reacted with disbelief that his patient was "awake" despite the Lupron (though he wasn't so awake that he could become hard), and that Michael's fantasies had switched so suddenly toward adults.

After six months, Fedoroff decided to cut Michael's dose of Lupron by half. Wakefulness increased. Erections, though fleeting, became possible. Fantasies stayed focused on adult women. He began to date. Any thoughts of children were like vestiges, easily put behind him. Recently, he told me, he'd played with his young nieces on the floor. "Not once did I have a deviant thought for any of them."

He felt he could do without the Lupron altogether. Fedoroff wasn't yet ready to take this step. But he trusted Michael's reports, didn't think they were driven by the wish to get free of the drug, free of Fedoroff's watch, and to get back to pursuing kids. Fedoroff saw him as a possible test of his theory.

He wanted Michael to find an adult partner, to build a stable relationship. The second language should be given time to develop. Then the Lupron could be eliminated, the full force of eros restored to this man who had danced his tongue between his daughter's legs with the ardor of love.

IN a statement Faith made to the police, which I discovered late in my time with Roy, I read that some of the touching, through clothes, began when she was in the second grade. Roy continued to insist that there had been nothing even suggestive of desire until she was eleven, until after that day at the shore. Faith's father, when I asked about the police statement, seemed unsure when to date the beginning of Roy's crimes. So I asked myself the obvious: Had the taint of recent times distorted Faith's vision of the past? Had Roy's propositions and his groping stained what had once been innocent? But I wondered, too, if I could believe anything he told me. Had he been lying from behind a veil of agonized introspection? Weren't child molesters often the most deft, the most subtle manipulators? Or was I posing the wrong kind of question? Was the sort of touching she described—a hand on her seven-year-old bottom, through pants—ever innocent?

With extreme reserve, Liddle fought to impose control. After their time in the tall grass and after their introductions, the men, at his direction, lifted loose-leaf binders from the floor beside their chairs. The blue-eyed poet who'd taken his brother and daughter to a motel room, and the white-haired retiree who'd fondled his grandniece—they owned the type of binder whose leatherette cover closes with a zipper. So did most of the others, as though this style could make a binder look like a briefcase and elevate their being here.

The binders were filled with the homework the men had done and the handouts they'd been given, with "Feelings Journals" and instructional sheets on techniques like "Thought Broadcasting": "If you get a deviant thought, imagine that your thought is being broadcast from your mind over a loudspeaker system."

There was, too, "Punishment Scene": "When you get a deviant thought, put your mind on fast forward to the part where you are held accountable for your actions."

And "Aversive Scene": "When you get a deviant thought, you begin to think about something that you find disgusting, e.g., Brussels sprouts. Or you could think about an experience that you don't like, e.g., going to the dentist."

Back in the 1970s, Liddle's boss told me, when the field of child-molester treatment was just developing, the prevailing strategy was psychodynamic—profound insight into the disinterred past was supposed to eliminate deviant desire. Mostly, it didn't, and by the early eighties, therapy shifted toward behavior modification. Offenders were instructed to inhale noxious odors during illicit fantasies. This brought success, but the success didn't last. Men plunged back into old longings. So cognitive-behavioral approaches, like Liddle's, took hold.

His sessions could seem more like classes in coping skills than anything that could be called treatment. The pragmatic and trite had replaced the penetrating and profound: thoughts of Brussels sprouts to quell deep-rooted need. Yet there were studies to suggest that the practical could displace the dark, that the trite was somehow profound, that the method might cut recidivism—which wasn't as high as people tended to imagine—by more than one-third.

Liddle asked the group to open their binders to a handout on "dynamic risk factors." He called on the white-haired man to read aloud, and the retiree, who liked to reminisce about how, when he was a boy, the probation building had been an ice factory, droned through definitions for the nine factors, from "negative social groups" to "distorted attitudes" to "victim access." These were to be recognized and avoided. "Intimacy deficits" was another factor that required awareness, caution, rectifying. And complexity lay quietly within this category: if loneliness was unsafe, then molesting involved reaching out for love.

Roy sat with his binder on his lap. His notebook was the thickest of any in the circle. He tried to think of the course as "a normal college class," to convince himself that diligence would guarantee graduation. Not only did he have the jumbo zippered binder with labeled dividers that he brought to group; he had another that he kept at home. He threw away nothing. He kept every page of evidence that he did everything Liddle asked.

On those pages were notes about "positive self-talk," a method to help the men keep themselves from feeling that they had nothing to lose. Roy was lucky in this regard. He had, for one thing, his job. His boss told me how his own wife felt about Roy: their children were grown, but she would have him in their house even if kids happened to be around. "That," his boss said, "is the confidence he gives you." Roy had plenty to lose, and still, driving over bridges, he fantasized about swerving through the rails. Thirty-five years of probation. He fantasized about the fall through the air, the descent through the water, the finality of it. Most of the others had the weekly circle of chairs and little else.

The pages were covered, as well, with notes on "maladaptive coping responses" and "adaptive coping responses." If the men woke in the middle of the night having had a deviant dream, what they should never do is lie there, touch themselves. They should get out of bed and get themselves a glass of milk. It was as though they were to swallow purity before returning to the danger of sleep.

Roy was doing well in Liddle's eyes. When Liddle asked for a definition and example of an "SUD," a "seemingly unimportant decision," Roy answered perfectly. It was like that with everything. His "action plans"—his applications to do what his probation restrictions did not permit—were composed at length and neatly typed out. When his sister gave birth, he put in a request to visit her over the state line. He was thorough in anticipating all the potential problems. "What if my brother-in-law's friends show up with their children?" he wrote. "What if my brother-in-law's brother came with his two girls and they were running through the house from room to room? I would say my good-byes and leave." His request was granted.

He applied for more and more freedoms, and they were given more and more often. He was allowed to take his fiancée bowling, to take her to the movies, to fly kites with her at the town beach. He asked to perform music at a local bar, which filled Liddle with fear. The bar didn't attract underage girls, but the therapist envisioned admirers and temptation: Roy picking up a strange woman and this leading—by way of eros unleashed—to his unraveling, his reoffending. Liddle refused the request, but intimated that, if Roy continued to show control, he might be performing soon.

And Roy applied to host a reception after his wedding to the bookkeeper. He applied to honeymoon down South. The problem with the reception was that the catering hall would be holding more than one event, and at the others, girls might be among the guests. "What if we are outside taking pictures and I need to go in and use the men's room? Since my brother is the best man, I would ask him to come with me so I was not walking through the building or the hallways alone."

ROY'S new wife wore white socks on her shoeless feet, blue jeans, a blue sweatshirt. It was a Friday night, and they had just finished their ritual Friday dinner: pizza and eggplant sandwiches. Now they sat close on their new couch, her feet tucked beneath her. Outside, on the windows, the shutters were adorned with quaint carvings. The house, his house, which she'd moved into, was pristine. The wood floors gleamed, the matching end tables were polished and bare. All felt at once irreproachable and ephemeral.

She was a few years older than Roy, but young-looking and slim, with brown bangs and a smile that held the endearing hint of an overbite. On their first date—three months after his arrest but before his plea, so that probation's restrictions and Liddle's rulings on his action plans didn't yet determine what he could and could not do—they'd flown his purple-and-aqua stunt kite. They laughed, on the couch, remembering the way it had yanked and dragged her down the beach. Besides the kites and the movies and the bowling, they'd gone for long walks, and he'd confided in her about his crime. "I've talked to her about everything," he said, as I sat with them. "I've talked to her about my thoughts when I was committing. I told her, 'If you're uncomfortable you can tell me. If you don't want to see me anymore you can tell me. But I have to be honest with you, I have to be.'"

"In my heart," she said, "I don't think he was this monster he was portrayed as in the paper." She was thinking of the articles in the small newspaper of his suburban town at the time of his arrest. "I didn't know what to believe. I couldn't believe the charges."

She described the plaque he'd won at work for most valuable employee of the year. "Who is Roy?" she asked, and answered herself, "He's very responsible. He's very kind. Very much like a little boy. Very playful. Very sincere."

On the night of the Fourth of July, they had gone to the shoreline park not far from his house and set a gargantuan kite aloft: the one he had outfitted with strobes. From high in the darkness it throbbed beams of orange and green and indigo down through the blue-black to color the sand.

They shifted closer to each other on the couch. She remembered, "One of the nicest things he ever said to me was that when he met me God was giving him a second chance."

He recalled her once telling him, "'When we go out flying, it's like an entire new day.'"

Her voice, as they spoke, was tender yet never fully surrendered to emotion. She could sound, at moments, utterly clearheaded and almost managerial, as though she had accounted and planned for every aspect of the past and future. But just before their wedding, Roy had talked in group about the meeting they'd had with her family priest, who was going to marry them. They told him about Roy's crime. The priest asked if she was really prepared for a life with a convicted child molester serving thirty-five years probation. "All of a sudden she was crying hysterically."

"I think," she said now on the couch, "I know Roy well enough to be sure he won't ever do that again. I think things just got out of hand." She wanted to take a special training course that would allow her to become an ancillary, probation-approved supervisor for her husband. This would give them a bit more freedom. And she felt it would teach her how to be on guard, how to save him. "I want to be able to recognize the signs, to know what to look for," she said. "People can stumble."

Then her voice sharpened severely. "To this day, I can't understand how he could write crap like that to a little girl. I tell him that all the time."

"She does," he mumbled, his soft face looking as though he'd been struck. "She does."

HIS fantasies emerged during a polygraph test. The men usually took the lie detector twice a year. The most incisive part sometimes came not when the machine was running but, beforehand, when anxiety was unbearable and the subject was asked to fill out a long questionnaire. During this section Roy confessed to thinking about Faith.

He'd said the same to me, more than once. "How do you turn it off? How do you turn off the thoughts that got you in so much trouble? Those conversations she had with her friend, they're still vivid in my mind. I'd be lying to you to tell you I'm not sexually aroused. Even at this point." And the thoughts, he felt, were "burned" into him by the group sessions themselves, by his being forced every week to walk the mazelike corridors and enter the windowless room and sit in the circle of chairs.

To Roy, the sessions offered no relief. After the discussions of dynamic risk factors and SUDs, Liddle tended to ask the men what deviant thoughts they'd had during the week just past. In over a year with the group, I never once heard the men speak more than a few words about desiring the young. "If we talked in there about what was really going through our minds," the poet once told me, "we'd all be wearing ankle bracelets." And Liddle didn't press. In response to the few words that were spoken, he quickly reviewed "thought broadcasting." Liddle, Roy said, "asks for deviant fantasy but he doesn't really want it."

The therapist talked with me about eliciting candor—but a candor that was delicately calibrated. Wrenching confessions, he felt, could destroy the composure he wanted to instill in the men. Too much honesty could stoke illicit fantasies. The men were forbidden to talk with one another outside the meetings. Liddle wished to "build up their sense of decency" and teach them to believe in their own capacity for restraint. In the windowless room, he allowed nothing to breach the atmosphere of control.

Roy had never so much as given the group any detail about the content of Faith's online talks with her friend. He had never really told his story. To imply that she'd played any small part in what had happened was forbidden. To call any attention to the fact that she had walked toward his computer when he'd invited her to see what he wished to do—this would have been the ultimate sin. In the back room, there were child victims and adult perpetrators. Nothing even slightly more nuanced was permitted, for fear that the men would justify their crimes to themselves. The men were trained to come down on each other for the faintest sign of deflecting responsibility. Roy kept his memories to himself.

Then, soon after the polygraph test, and after his wife had applied to be trained as an ancillary supervisor, it came out—indirectly, during a discussion in group—that she and Roy hadn't told her parents about his crime. Liddle worried that, had she completed the training without this deception emerging, they could have been at any sort of family function with her parents, and, if young girls were around, her priority would have been to keep Roy's secret rather than to tell her parents they had to leave. Despite being his entrusted supervisor, she might have allowed him to stay.

But the deception itself was even worse. Liddle saw a man in denial, a man failing the program's fundamental requirements of honesty and self-confrontation, a man who should have delivered, in group, a simple, undetailed admission of his fantasies, and who should have been clear about the situation with his in-laws. In the evasion of candor, Liddle sensed the threat of anarchy.

His fear was compounded by an answer on another questionnaire: Roy was having sex with his wife several times each week. This seemed to Liddle a sign of excessive urgency. Roy told me that he was sexually satisfied, that his wife was taking care of all his needs. Liddle mentioned to me that he was considering trying to convince Roy to take medication to reduce, though not eliminate, his sex drive. There would be no legal requirement that Roy agree. But Liddle's influence over what he could and could not do, over the rest of his life, might persuade him.

The therapist held off on medication. He limited himself to taking away Roy's privileges—the visits to his family, the bowling, the movies, the kite-flying. The prospect of performing his music was now beyond discussion. Except for work, Roy would remain inside his house. Eros would be kept within.

ONE night, shortly before his privileges were taken away, Roy and his wife had launched a vast, luminous gold-and-red kite at the town beach. Usually after dusk the beach was empty. But a group of kids—"a mob," it seemed to him—came running toward them, boys and girls who looked between the ages of four and twelve. By his agreement with Liddle and the probation department, he was simply supposed to tell the kids to keep their distance, to tell them they might get tangled in the heavy lines. The mere presence of the underage didn't mean he had to leave the waterfront. But everything had begun at the edge of the water. The words of Faith's mother had come with the sound of the surf. And now he panicked. He handed the unwieldy lines to his wife and, whether dreading some imagined probationary infraction or terrified of something inside himself, he raced away.

He rushed for the waist-high fence that divided the beach from the parking lot. But he couldn't get his bearlike body over it. He got stuck, sitting on the wire, crushing it, caught between the shore and the pavement. He couldn't get free.

PART IV

THE DEVOTEE

WHEN SHE WAS A GIRL, LAURA AND HER FRIENDS rode their horses through the Pennsylvania countryside, rode Western and bareback, rode through woods and cornfields. The woods seemed to belong to no one. The cornfields churned around them like windswept lakes. They galloped through the afternoons till it was time for dinner. Her father was a truck driver. The family, with five kids, lived on a scrap of farmland with a pond, a few cows, some corn.

She had an implausible dream. It was something she kept to herself. She wanted to be a psychiatrist, dreamed of it even before she reached high school. "Oh gosh," she remembered decades later, "I always thought that the way we think and behave is so fascinating. It is so complex. I thought what a great thing to be able to do, to figure that out. Every kid growing up knows what a doctor and a lawyer is, but to me it was just like, who would want to be a doctor or a lawyer? I want to be a psychiatrist—wouldn't that be intriguing! In high school I would go to the library and read. Some Freud. A lot of self-help books. Some Jung."

No one in her family had gone to college. Few of the girls she spent time with had plans to. She knew her family couldn't afford it. She didn't think she was smart enough, anyway. She was fast in her typing course, fast and accurate; she figured she'd be a secretary. Behind psychiatry, her second fantasy was to be a model. People said she should be. She had a cascade of blond hair, full lips, eyes that were a crystal blue. But she knew she was too short. She thought: I'm going to get married and work in an office, because that is realistic.

In her junior year, she started going to parties with a good-looking, weed-smoking senior. He'd been staring at her from the end of one of the long tables in their home economics class. They married as soon as she graduated. He joined the Air Force; she got pregnant. She followed him wherever he was stationed, from Delaware to England to Texas, caring for their son, sometimes babysitting for extra money, sometimes working at the PX on base. In San Antonio, she found a job as a secretary for a company that made eyeglasses. About college and psychiatry, she felt the way she always had: "That is for other people. That is somebody else's dream."

One wet Friday morning, as she drove to work, her Mustang ran out of gas on a highway that looped around the city. The pavement was slick, and the traffic was stalled.

A thousand and more miles away, in Manhattan, Ron sketched scenes that sold liquor: couples falling in love, parties at the beach, gatherings in a loft, excursions on a yacht. He was in advertising, an art director; he conjured billboards and posters. He created the concepts and, with a photographer, cast the models. He searched for young women to fill his tableaux of love, of high spirits, of sophistication, women who would infuse any viewer with longing and envy.

He had grown up in Queens, in neighborhoods of small apartment buildings and little clapboard houses with dormers and low stoops. In backyards of concrete and on the pavement of the street, he and his friends had sprayed one another with water guns, played stickball and roller-skate hockey. They drew giant chalk squares with numbered boxes and dead-man zones for games of skully—they knelt on the asphalt and flicked their bottle caps till their mothers, leaning out from windows and shrieking their names, called them home for dinner. La-Guardia Airport was close by. The gates and runways were unguarded; they staged war games throughout the terminals and on the tarmac.

But one afternoon he found himself riding his bicycle furtively along tree-lined streets. He sped around corners with the sense that everyone, every adult and everyone his own age, was staring through the back of his head, seeing what he was imagining. At the library, he jammed his red one-speed into the rack, and, eyes averted, he stepped past the librarian and sidled between the dark wooden tables.

ABOUT that Friday morning, Laura told things this way: "I said good-bye to my husband while he was sleeping in bed, and I left the house and got into my car. I was in a hurry, and that gauge wasn't very accurate. So I was like, I think I have enough to get to work, I should be all right, I'll get gas on my lunch hour. Everything was backed up on the freeway. My engine died, and I pumped and cursed and got it going again just long enough to steer onto the side. I got out, and this lady, this rich, classy lady, pulled over in a Lincoln. She told me she could take me to the nearest station, which was right off the next exit. The man inside told me to leave a three-dollar deposit for the can.

"The lady was really friendly. She said she would take me back. She dropped me off, and I thanked her, and I walked around to the side of my car where the gas tank was. The traffic was moving along by then, and I realized it was too dangerous, because I was standing slightly out into the lane. I hesitated. I knew it was too dangerous, but I didn't know what to do. I hesitated for that second, having those thoughts, and then I got hit.

"All I remember is being thrown through the air. And then when I woke up I heard all these people around me, and I was laying there on the side of the road, and I was trying to get up, and they were like, 'It's okay, it's okay,' and I was thinking my legs were broken, in my mind my legs were broken, and I grabbed onto a lady's coat, and I said, 'Please help me.'

"She told me an ambulance was coming. I really didn't know what had happened. They put me in those inflatable things so you don't bleed to death. And then I was in the emergency room, and the doctors were coming in, and they were touching and twisting my legs, and I was saying to myself, I was struck and my legs were broken, I was struck and my legs were broken. They kept twisting. It seemed like forever, like hours and hours. Oh my gosh I was in such pain. Why were they doing this? It went on and on, and I never looked down, and then one doctor stood over me, and he said, 'I need to tell you that your legs were severely crushed, and you need to go into surgery right away.'

"They put a mask over my mouth and told me to take three breaths. That was it until I woke up again. And then I would not look down. The doctors said I almost died. They said they had never seen anyone's blood pressure fall so low and still live, that it was a miracle I was still there, if it had been any longer I would have bled to death. I couldn't even look. Everything was a fog. I was so heavily medicated I would go in and out of consciousness. I remember somebody saying, 'I cannot believe she has no other injury or trauma on her body.' All I had was a couple of stitches up here on my head and a black-and-blue mark under my eye. Nothing else was wrong. They did all the tests they could, and there was nothing.

"I never watched them change the dressings. They said, 'You're going to have to do this yourself,' but I wouldn't pay any attention. They did it twice a day, and I would shut my eyes or keep them somewhere else in the room. They had told me right away after the surgery, but you can't grasp that. You can't one day be walking and the next—you can't accept it. You can't face it. You know it intellectually, but you block it off. For two weeks I never once looked down.

"They had told me they couldn't save them, but the first time I acknowledged it was when they sent me to rehab, because I had to get out of bed. Yet even still, even though I knew it was true, I was so drugged up it was almost a dream.

"And I remember Scott—that's my son—asking, 'Will Mommy's legs grow back?' and my mom saying, 'No, honey, they won't.' He didn't say anything. And I remember lots of people there; the guy who drove the ambulance and someone who saw the accident came to see how I was doing. I remember the look on my husband's face. And I remember all the flowers, so many flowers they overfilled the room. I wished I had died. I thought, Why didn't they just let me die? Because one morning I was walking, and when I looked down my legs were gone."

• • •

LATER Ron would wonder if he'd been made an unknowing subject of a secret army experiment. He would warn himself he was being paranoid, then wonder if he was being perfectly rational, given the sorts of things the army and the government were capable of carrying out. He saw himself, too, as suffering from what he called "the Godzilla syndrome"—radiation from nuclear testing had skewed his psyche.

But on that boyhood afternoon when he made his swift way past the librarian, he was simply terrified. He picked out the volumes of the encyclopedias and piled them on a table.

His first crush had come years earlier, when he was five years old. The woman ran a clothing shop with her sister, a few blocks from his home. Walking with his mother, he tugged and schemed daily to steer her in that direction. Whenever he succeeded, he gazed between the dresses and bras in the window to glimpse his first love. She had black hair and wore stubby black shoes—like a nun, he thought. One of the shoes, with a higher heel and thicker sole than the other, was built to compensate for a short leg.

It was the leg, a consequence of polio, that mesmerized him. By the time of his trip to the library, Ron had taken to erasing or scratching out limbs on pictures of women. In the encyclopedias he hoped for something less makeshift, less messy, more real. He chose the volumes holding articles on amputation. He picked, too, the ones that included polio and any other crippling disease he could name. He searched for articles on rehabilitation, thinking that this subject might provide the photographs or illustrations he'd anticipated. But, except for a picture of an iron lung, he found nothing. The images had been razored out. It was his first clue that he wasn't completely alone.

The clue didn't have much effect. As a teenager, he went out with the normal in body, while his yearnings were for the disabled. One of his father's favorite words seemed to be "gimp"; he certainly wasn't going to open up to his parents. An older girl, legs in braces—another polio victim—propelled herself through the neighborhood on crutches. He knew when she would be coming home from school, knew where she lived. He made sure to cross her path, to pass by her house; he never approached her. And a girl with cerebral palsy went to his own school, where each day she was tormented, called spastic and "Judy Cooty." He tried to defend her, but that was all. For dates he chose the kinds of girls his friends desired. Pressed against them, "I closed my eyes and imagined that they didn't have a leg or an arm."

He went to college, studied to be an architect but immersed himself in fine art, married a woman he'd met in a drawing class, felt profoundly allied with her, loved the fact that as they walked through the Louvre they both revered Gericault over da Vinci, the *Raft of the Medusa* over the *Mona Lisa*, but blamed her for the feeling that there was nothing profound—that there was almost nothing at all—between them in bed. Soon they divorced. And meanwhile he began his career in advertising, his celebration of quotidian beauty, his evocation of Everyman's ideal and elicitation of Everyman's longing. He drew and cast and produced perfect scenes populated by perfect women, who could stir in him no wanting, whose beauty to him was abstract, who made him feel dead.

BENEATH the wish to die lay determination. Laura was driven by devotion to her five-year-old son, "the cutest blond-haired curly kid you ever saw." And she was driven by the staff. They seemed to have only one focus, to be capable of only one concern: to get her onto prosthetics, to get her walking, to fit her back inside her life. In the rehabilitation rooms of the hospital they strapped her to weights, pushed her to strengthen her upper body, taught her to understand the movements her legs could still perform. Both legs had been amputated about ten inches below her hips.

Almost half her body had vanished. She felt alone not only in the world that she knew awaited her but even within the hospital walls. She was surrounded, at rehabilitation, by patients at least twice her age, victims of stroke and degenerative disease. "I'm twenty-five years old," she recalled thinking. "How many years do I have to live this way? How many years are left? How am I going to raise my child? How am I going to walk? How am I going to have sex? Who is— All this stuff is running through my head every day from the minute I wake up, and every morning it's, 'Eight o'clock! Get your mat!' I'm crumbling inside, I'm crushed to the very core, and they're saying, 'Eight o'clock! Get your mat! Eight o'clock! Get your mat!'"

There was no psychological counseling to speak of. She heard no answers to most of the questions that woke and whispered and screamed with her own waking, nothing beyond meaningless reassurances from those who knew her: she was strong, she'd always had spirit, she would get through this. Through to what? What did "through" mean? This wasn't temporary. She wasn't traveling backward in time. Could she? Was she? Are Mommy's legs going to grow back?

She obeyed the eight o'clock orders, wheeled herself to rehab. Prosthetics were made and fitted; she steadied herself on the parallel bars. "'Pick up your right leg slowly,'" they instructed. She picked it up, put it down. Sensation traveled to her stump. "'Pick up the foot again.'" And it was as though there were a foot—vaguely. The prosthetic communicated, dimly, to what remained of the limb. She registered the surface underneath, its degree of hardness, flatness, reliability.

But this was not the ad that ran on TV, the one with the silky playground basketball player lifting off for a jump shot on his artificial legs. His amputations were below the knee. For ease of adapting, for fullness of function, for balance and mobility, the player's body was closer to whole than it was to Laura's. And there was nothing magical about the prosthetics she'd been given, nothing bionic, little of what people imagined science could offer. It wasn't that she'd been given anything substandard. It was that the miraculous didn't exist. The legs were limited in what they could be commanded to do. Technology couldn't replace muscles and nerves. It could allow for bending but it couldn't replicate the complexity of a knee, and it couldn't provide anything more than crude control over the artificial joint.

"I would give anything in this world for my legs back, except for my son," she wrote in her journal. The journal came with sketches and sayings on some of its pages. In one of the drawings, a nude goddess, whose body appeared to end at the knees, was borne aloft by a population of devoted, unclothed worshippers. One of the aphorisms went like this: "In truth we talk only to ourselves, but sometimes we talk loud enough that others may hear us."

She didn't talk loudly, not when it came to the questions that whispered and screamed. She just held herself upright on the parallel bars. She just picked up a foot and put it down, repeated and repeated this, then did the same with the other. She took a step. She took two. She made it to the end of the bars. There possibility ended, as though she had come to the edge of a cliff. There life itself seemed to end. Capability, what meager ration she now had, was cut off.

She managed to turn around. A step, another, a third, a fourth. To the end, the cliff, and back again, hands clinging on, hands for balance, hands to keep her from falling like a plank, hands like a baby's on furniture as it learns to walk, but she without a baby's future, she with this body—was *this* a body?—forever. Her son was sometimes there visiting, watching. Thinking back to that time, she couldn't remember what was said between them. It seemed they hadn't spoken at all. "Maybe there wasn't a lot to say."

A doctor had complimented what existed of her thighs: the fitting of prosthetics wouldn't be difficult. But the fabricated limbs cut agonizingly into her groin. They had to be reshaped. Then the swelling of her stumps went down. More fitting, followed by more pain, more rounds of adjustments. And all the while, despite the pain, she stepped back and forth, back and forth along the parallel bars, exhausting herself so completely that sleep came by six o'clock.

She woke to the same truths that had dominated the day before, the same long void when she looked down, the same long void of years in front of her, woke eventually at home when she was discharged. A visiting nurse taught her to use a portable toilet until she could lever herself onto the regular one. Within two weeks she taught herself to pull and writhe her body into and out of the tub, so her husband no longer had to lift her in and out. Having mastered the dogged movements of a walker, she tried crutches in their driveway. To keep her upright, her husband walked behind her, bracing her with a strap.

He wheeled her, one night, into a bar where a friend of theirs was performing. "The band was real good," she recounted in her journal. "We ate tamales and drank beer. I was watching everyone dance to the country music Rusty sang, and I felt I would give anything to be up there on the dance floor. It hurt me to see everyone dancing. I cried the whole way home. It felt like someone tore my heart out." On a later evening, for her husband's birthday, when she could approximate a walk on her prosthetics, they went to another bar to hear another band. As they were leaving, making their drunken way across the parking lot, one of her legs fell off.

"He never talks about my accident," she wrote. "We seem to not be able to communicate. I think he is keeping it all bottled up inside. I guess it's the military way or else he doesn't have any feelings."

He had always liked to stay out with his friends, on his own and late; now he stayed out more often and later. And there were nights he didn't keep things to himself at all. He blamed her for what had happened, for being careless, for letting the gas tank go empty, for stepping around to the side of the car. After a night of drinking at their house, with her mother visiting along with friends from his tour in England, he took a rifle from a closet. He declared that he was driving over to kill the woman who had done this to her. They had the police report, knew her name and address. The woman had never so much as called; she'd never even sent a card. Rifle in hand, he raged until their guests restrained him.

There was sex. But it was she, as much as her husband, who avoided it, couldn't bear it. She was a woman whose prosthetics sometimes farted out pockets of air as she stood up; a woman who rode to her sessions of physical therapy on a special bus filled with retarded children; a woman who was stared at constantly; a woman who was told in a kindly voice by her neighbor at the mailboxes, "I don't know if I could deal with that"—with having Laura's body, with being what Laura was.

Laura asked to see her X-rays. "I want proof," she confided in her journal, "that the doctors had to do what they had to do. I know it will really hurt, but I want to see it for myself. Maybe it will help me accept."

A doctor clipped up the images, clicked on the white light. "The knees were all broken in half," she wrote. "The bones were all broken in half. There was a dark spot on the right one. He said the bone was missing when I arrived there. It must have been on the side of the road.

"To look at those X-rays realizing that those were my legs brought a feeling of such great loss. He told me if they had been his they would have come off. He said a vascular surgeon was called to see if they could be saved, and there was no way. Not only were the bones broken up but all the tissue and muscle and cartilage was ruined. He told me he would show me the photos, but I refused. Do not look back but move ahead now. He said you're young and pretty and have a complete and fulfilling life ahead of you."

Desolate, determined, exhilarated, she walked away from the X-rays. She walked away, clinging to his words. But they evaporated, turned fast to nothing. They were a trick, a lie. "I was disgusting. No man could ever want me," she said. "My whole life I was told I was pretty. Now what do I have? Now that I don't have that, now that I'm revolting, what do I have?"

For resilience she relied not on the doctor's words but on a patient she saw in physical therapy. The woman was paralyzed from the waist down. Legs in braces and body supported by a therapist, she was walking—in a sense. But it was only an exercise. It was nothing she would ever do on her own. Her legs, Laura thought with a piercing satisfaction, were utterly useless. They would be that way forever, while Laura was capable of walking by herself.

For resilience this was what she had: "There are people worse off than me."

A year after losing her legs, she overdosed on Valium and nearly succeeded in killing herself.

IN Berlin, in the years between world wars, there was an artist who began in advertising. Hans Bellmer designed campaigns for household products and then, as the Nazis took power, gave up all commercial work and concentrated on building two female dolls, almost life-sized, made from papier-mâché and plaster, metal and wood. The limbs could be bent and twisted. The heads could tilt and pivot. A second pair of legs could be attached to a central ball joint on one of the dolls. Extra breasts and buttocks and pelvises could be appended. Body parts could be removed.

He photographed his dolls in poses of distortion and dismemberment, then gave the pictures, in the form of a tiny self-published book, to his beautiful seventeen-year-old cousin, whose arrival in his life, not as a lover he touched but as the embodiment of desire, had inspired the invention of the figures, the arrangement and rearrangement, the taking apart and putting back together of what he had made, the capturing with his camera. The cousin managed to give the photographs to the French surrealist poet André Breton. And Breton published them in his magazine, *Minotaure*.

It was the start of a career that took Bellmer to live in Paris and put him in a circle with Man Ray, Max Ernst, Marcel Duchamp. His method was obsessive. His output was minuscule, his life impoverished. He drew, he made collages, but three decades later, approaching his own death, he was still working with one of his two dolls, finding new ways to transfigure the body he had formed. Next to the other artists in his group, he was unknown, invisible. But those who discovered him were haunted: he took them inside a more harrowing subconscious than the other surrealists seemed willing to confront.

A nude girl, both childish and fully developed, lies sprawled near the bottom of a wooden staircase. It is one of Bellmer's dolls with a pink bow in her hair and high, prominent breasts. She seems, in the photograph, to have been pushed down the stairs; one leg is missing at the hip. And it looks like violence has been done to her before, that her other knee has been broken in the past: rope, crudely knotted, seems to brace it. An arm, too, has been severed. Shadows mottle her skin, and the bottom banister of the stair rail obscures half of her face. The fingers of her remaining hand peek from behind the banister— the fingers are both trying to grab on, to stop her fall, and waving, beckoning the viewer of the photograph, who feels himself to be standing in the shadows that deepen at the foreground of the picture. Bangs cover her forehead: she is innocent. Her chin rests between her breasts, and her mouth is slightly open: she is seductive. She looks, at once, as though she has been knocked unconscious and as though she is sleeping, sated. And she looks aroused, wanting. Her belly protrudes, and the uptilted slit of her vagina occupies the center of the frame.

"Fit joint to joint, testing the ball-joints by turning them to their maximum position in a childish pose," he wrote in an essay that accompanied his first book of photographs, his words sometimes taking the form of instructions to himself—a how-to for fabricating and disfiguring a doll. "Gingerly follow the hollows, sampling the pleasures of curves, losing oneself in the clamshell of the ear, creating beauty and also distributing the salt of deformation a bit vengefully." His work was driven by the wish to explore his own—and the viewer's—longing, but also by the ambition to expose the yearnings of the girl. "Don't stop short of the interior," he instructed himself. "Lay bare suppressed girlish thoughts." His images should reveal, inside the figure, the violent battle "between desire and its interdiction."

Another photograph is taken from behind. A sleeveless and flimsy undergarment, held up by a single shoulder strap, covers part of the girl's back. Her head is turned; her chin lies hidden against her right shoulder; her lips nearly brush the strap; she gazes at the camera. The back half of her head is gone, cut away. Luxuriant curls of hair grow from her open skull and fall profligately past her neck and down her spine. Her body is bare except for the undergarment, which reaches only to her waist. But there isn't much body left. She has no arms. The socket of one shoulder is ragged. The flesh of one leg has been stripped from the limb itself. The other leg has been replaced by a twig-thin mechanism with a joint at the knee that looks like a minimalist prosthetic. The round buttocks sit atop these legs, voluptuous. A bit of their paper skin is cracked and eroding, making them look somehow all the more sensual and obscene, all the more provocative. The surface of her face is cracked and scratched as well. A bruise adorns the corner of one eye, and she gazes back out of that corner, fearful, inviting, anticipating that the viewer will approach her, assault her, take her from behind. Her shadow blackens one wall. The walls around her are tight. She is wedged into one corner of the room. Even if she wanted to escape, there would be no way.

There are those who have seen Bellmer's art as a reaction against Nazism, who have decided that his portraits of the female body were meant as a protest against Nazism's reverence for physical perfection. Yet he scorned all political and moral aims. "Pulp writers, magicians, and confectioners used to have that secret something, that beautiful sweet which was called nonsense and that brings joy," he wrote, aligning his aesthetic with theirs. "They dispensed with that unhappiness normally associated in my experience with useful intentions, and revealed the mysteries of roads less traveled by." For Bellmer, the sweet and the harrowing—inseparable—were the path to revelation.

The doll, doe-eyed, leans back against a wall, oblivious to the fact that the skin of her stomach has been torn off, uncovering the hollow within, as though she has been disemboweled. Both arms are gone from their sockets. A leg has been lost. The doe eyes gaze slightly upward, unalarmed, receptive. The nose has a cute curve.

The doll, in another image, is reduced to the head and chest, nothing below that, and rests on the edge of a decrepit washbasin. Doe eyes have been replaced by wide, blank eyeballs. Her bangs are a pair of wispy spikes. The scalp is balding. Four perfectly spherical breasts protrude from the upper torso: two from the shoulders, one from the center of the chest, one from the side of the ribcage. The invitation, the terror, the innocence that animate the faces in the other photographs are absent. All expression is absent. Not only the eyes but the entire face is vacant. The girl is ravaged, dead, resilient only in the sexuality that is so aggressively present in the four breasts. The way her half-torso sits balanced on the rim of the chipped basin makes her look all the more assaulted, abandoned.

Yet beauty infuses the picture, just as it does all the others: the beauty of starkness, of the interplay between the texture of walls and the texture of flesh, the beauty of things seen in all their mute strangeness, the beauty of the bewildering, never explained but always illuminated. A doll, headless, with two sets of legs and groins, sprawled on a mattress in what seems to be the aftermath of making love to itself; a doll, headless, with two sets of legs and groins, sprawled on a field of dry grass in what seems to be the aftermath of rape; a doll without arms and only half of one leg suspended high in a tree, the photograph taken from below so that she floats, ethereal, in a blanched sky; a doll diminished to several distorted buttocks, nothing more, and cast in gold—all are suffused by the light of Bellmer's ardent focus, his thrall, his love.

In middle age, Bellmer began an affair with an artist and writer fourteen years younger, Unica Zurn. She became his model and muse, a living doll. In a double-sided drawing, done in thread-thin white lines on black paper, Zurn stands, wearing a suit whose modest skirt reaches below her knees, with her hands folded demurely in front of her pelvis. That is the image on one side of the paper. On the reverse side, she is down on all fours, her skirt short and pleated. She wears striped socks and Mary Janes—the girlish shoes he often put on his dolls as he posed them. The drawing holds a single element of collage, a pink hair bow. Her face, turned to the side, almost grazes the floor as she peers at a child's glass marble, her fingers poised to touch it. The marble was symbolic to him: "a view of its interior allowed one to observe the frozen ecstasy of its spirals." On hands and knees, both animal and child, Zurn gazes into the spirals of her own erotic being, transfixed and tempted to go further.

For a photograph, he bound her torso and buttocks tightly, asymmetrically, over and over and over with twine. She curls on a bed so that, from the back, her head, arms, legs are all out of view. What's left for the camera are uncanny, anarchic risings of flesh extruding around the string, a crazed flowering of flesh, an abstract sculpture made from the most figurative of objects, the human body, an attempt to reach beneath the conscious to the unnamable.

But while she was model and muse, Zurn had her own voice. Her novella *Dark Spring* was, she said, "the erotic life of a little girl based on my own childhood." Ten and eleven and twelve years old as the story unfolds, the girl fantasizes about kidnappers binding her fiercely and raping her with a knife, penetrating her with the blade. She is "honored" by all they do.

"Scenes of madness, of torture, of ecstasy were drawn by Bellmer with the sensitivity of a musician, the precision of an engineer, the brusqueness of a surgeon," Zurn declared. "If we watch him at work, his hand seems weightless. One wants to know if it is tense against the paper, or if this pleasing line is a piece of sorcery from the void. . . . Whoever is sketched by him shares with him the abhorrence of self. It is impossible for me to render him greater praise."

The girl and her violent fantasies, the adult and her urge to be annihilated through her lover's art—Zurn was the proof, in blood and muscle and brain, of Bellmer's vision of eros. But neither character nor author, it seemed, could survive the desire they had opened up in themselves. At the novella's end, the girl kills herself, and soon after the book was published, Zurn committed suicide exactly as her character does: jumping from a window, destroying her body on the ground below, leaving herself broken like one of Bellmer's dolls.

ON his lunch hour, between sketching scenes to sell liquor and hiring conventionally pretty women to inhabit them, Ron walked the city with his camera. Manhattan seemed a dreamscape dominated by the vertical: not only the buildings but the crowds of pedestrians formed a world that was relentlessly straight up and down. "A disabled person," he said, "is a break in that strict verticality, a diagonal in that mass."

He sought out the diagonals to photograph, taking the images, at first, covertly, aiming his lens swiftly on the streets. In one picture, a woman propels herself along the sidewalk amid a stream of shoppers, propels herself partly on legs with braces, partly on crutches. Her bare muscled arms in a sleeveless dress, her in-twisting feet in elegant shoes, her slender hips thrust outward by her skewed stride, her chest leaning, almost lunging far forward of her legs, the angles of body parts accentuated by the straightness of the crutches—the entire effect is of a mime or a dancer expressively bent, except that this figure is more bent and expressive than a healthy body could ever manage. She is sculptural: contorted, animated, allusive, mesmerizing.

Another photograph captures a crippled woman through eyes other than his own. His quick focusing and clicking was meant simply to record the woman as she maneuvered herself off a curb on crutches. But without intending to, he included in the frame an onlooker standing behind his subject. Ron's lens focuses in one direction, reverently, on the woman making her way off the sidewalk, while the bystander stares in the opposite direction, her eyes angling downward at the subject's lower legs, at the deformation or absence that is cut out of the frame, that the photograph does not reveal. The bystander's gaze is far from reverent. Her fingers touch her lips in horror.

His first love after his marriage came through his camera. He approached Elise on a crosstown bus, asked if she would consider posing. As a child she'd been one of the last in her hometown to contract polio. She'd been out of school, not feeling well, when the vaccine was given, and her parents had never bothered to have her inoculated. Now she was studying for a master's degree in social work. Petite, with high cheekbones and a dimpled chin, a small lush mouth and long lush hair, she wore steel braces on both useless legs.

He photographed her only once in almost a year. They spent their time enmeshed in each other's bodies, she comfortable in hers because he was so ardent with his, and immersed in debating the merits of his mainstream ambitions versus hers, after she graduated, to rehabilitate prisoners. She lived in the East Village, in her sister's apartment, on a block that served as a base for the Hell's Angels. A few of the gang surrounded him early on, grabbed him, asked if he was seeing Elise. "You mess her up and we'll kill you," one of them warned. Ron photographed her only once, because her face was almost always bruised, an eye sometimes black. Her husband beat her.

Though she stayed with her sister, she and her husband were still involved. Ron saw her when her husband traveled. Her husband never discovered the affair; the beatings weren't on Ron's account. Ron never knew the reason, knew only that Elise tolerated it, allowed it. He thought she believed it was what she had coming, as a cripple, that she believed she could do no better, felt she was lucky to have a husband at all. But he never tried to convince her to divorce, to be with him. Later, after they had drifted apart, he was desperate to find her, see her, persuade her. He called, but the phone was disconnected. He went to the apartment; the Hell's Angels told him the sisters had moved away. He assumed Elise was still married, but he kept searching. He tried to locate the sister. He called the bureau of prisons in Elise's home state, where he guessed Elise might have gone, and begged for a list of their social workers. He hired a private detective.

During their time together, he said, he had fallen for her "in a way that went far beyond my fascination." The word—

"fascination"—was the term men like Ron sometimes used, men drawn to the disabled. "The attraction," he remembered, "became this wonderful overlay to what we had." They had opened up to each other, she released by the improbable direction of his desire and he by holding, and being held fiercely by, a figure from his dreams. But he hadn't been ready, and his dream had disappeared, and the private detective could not find her. He hadn't been ready at all, not to be permanent and public with a woman who looked like she did. He was barely willing to admit what he wanted to himself. Clandestine, ashamed, his ambivalence seemed to have affirmed her shame, her feeling that her husband was her due. With her braces, her beauty, her black eyes, she was gone.

He went to two psychologists, and in their offices avoided the subject, the elemental aspect of himself, that had driven him to seek their help. With the first therapist he filled the sessions with the failings of his ex-wife. But the second seemed to intuit his evasions. He asked about the camera Ron always carried, wondered what he took pictures of. "And?" the therapist pressed gently. "And? And?"

He persisted until Ron confided everything, then asked Ron if he hurt anyone, if he hurt himself. So there was, the psychologist advised, no reason for self-reproach, no reason for reluctance. It was far from that simple. Yet the therapist's logic began to unburden him as he went on photographing and sleeping with women he met around the city.

Katherine had hooks for hands and one prosthetic leg—a pornographic fantasy, but there wasn't much between them in bed: "She would never take off her nightgown. She was a lot more inhibited about her body than Elise." It was her determination that enthralled him. She wanted to become an occupational therapist, but to be certified she had to lift an impossible weight. She went to court, proved the requirement unnecessary and prejudicial, got her license, and started her career. He remembered, too, the way she ate olives with pits when they went to a favorite Greek restaurant. "Not an easy thing for anyone to do gracefully," he laughed. "But somehow she did."

Melinda he met on the street while walking after lunch. She was with a friend who assumed that Ron, intruding himself and explaining that he wanted to do a portrait, was really interested in her. Melinda was, after all, just a paraplegic in a wheelchair. The friend volunteered that she had always wanted to be a model, that it would be great if he could take some head shots. He did a session for both of them, gave the pretty would-be model the pictures she needed, then focused his lens on the woman who entranced him.

Sylvia was South American, an accountant with a serene oval face, a close-mouthed smile, lustrous black hair. She sobbed uncontrollably after she and Ron first made love. Her legs, wasted by disease, could support her only with a lattice-work of steel bars and leather straps. She lived alone in a hotel, never spoke of family or friends, and when she visited Ron's apartment always tuned the radio to an oldies station. She wanted the love songs of earlier decades, the serenades of doo-wop. One day, when he called her, the woman at the hotel's front desk, who usually took his messages, asked him to come over. She told him, when he arrived, that his girlfriend had killed herself.

Elizabeth was the valedictorian of her Ivy League class, and Ron happened to hear her commencement address. "She was about as close as I expected to come to the ideal woman," he remembered. "She was smart, she was cute, and she had no legs." That evening after the graduation, he called the dorms, reached someone who knew her, learned that she had already left for the summer. But he was told, too, that she would be back for law school in the fall. He phoned her then, praised her speech, persuaded her to go out on a date. She met him at the campus gates with three of the university's football players standing beside her wheelchair.

The campus wasn't wheelchair-accessible, and a squad of athletes was assigned to carry her up stoops and bear her up flights of stairs. In this case, though, they were there for protection. What kind of creep or lunatic would want to date a woman with no legs? But when she met him, he seemed safe and sane enough. She told the players they could go. He wheeled her out the gates.

She had grown up in small Southern towns with an affliction that shortened her legs and froze her joints at the ankles, knees, hips. Twenty-some operations by the time she was thirteen—surgeons breaking bones, cutting tendons, reattaching ligaments—didn't bring mobility to her legs. Then a doctor suggested amputation; her real legs would never be any use to her, but she might walk with prosthetics. She went through another surgery, woke with her legs removed, and never could train herself to walk well on artificial limbs. She told Ron she didn't regret the amputation. She said that whenever she saw paraplegics with their legs, she thought only of their stupidity— they were burdened with so much meaningless weight.

Intellectual, imperious, self-sufficient, she captivated him, and after a few months together, he tried what he never had with any girlfriend. He possessed, by then, a degree of self-acceptance. The psychologist had helped, and so had finding a group of similar men, who called themselves "devotees." They met, as a kind of support group, at the home of a former Korean War pilot who had lately befriended a veteran of the

Algerian resistance. She'd blown off her legs while trying to blow up a French building.

What he tried was telling Elizabeth about his desire for the disabled and above all for amputees. She seemed incredulous, rapt, then grateful, released. She posed for him in ways that alluded to the erotic power she'd just discovered. In one portrait, her abbreviated body sits draped in red fabric: her stumps, covered in sheer black nylons and partially concealed in shadow, might easily be overlooked. But on second glance they emerge: paired secrets, half-hidden parts, objects of shame and allure, transfixing.

They married after he'd carried her up the three flights of stairs to his apartment for three years. "My friends were like a Greek chorus. Charlie Crane, who I lived with for two years, who I worked with for fifteen years, who I traveled with all the time, was absolutely rabid. He just flat-out said, 'Why would you want someone with no legs? I can't go out with you anymore. I don't want to deal with it, I can't deal with it, it's ugly.' Charlie's girlfriends, you could look through their heads, but they were tall and skinny. They had long legs and big breasts and blond hair."

Others kept their quiet distance and faded away. "They just didn't want to be seen with her. It just didn't fit the image they wanted." And Elizabeth was adept at making them uneasy. She insisted on wearing miniskirts and on never wearing prosthetics. At a Christmas party, as she sat on a couch with her stumps protruding, someone asked if she would cover herself with a blanket. For the beach she chose bikinis, never anything that even intimated an effort to conceal. She liked Ron to carry her across the sand to the water, to put her down at the edge of the surf. And in a car one intoxicated evening, she sent shudders through his friends by vaulting herself from the backseat into the front, launching her body like some sort of tree-jumping animal.

"You have to develop the same thick skin they have," he said about being with Elizabeth and the lovers who had come before her. "Society sees you like you're driving around in a junk car. A woman with a disability is like that. Everyone stares. And everyone wants to ask, 'Why are you with a defective person?'"

"WHEN people hear we split up, they think, This happened to you, so your husband left you. But I was the one who filed," Laura said. "He might have left me emotionally, but I was the one who filed for divorce. And that took a lot of guts. I had a son to raise and no legs and no education except a high school diploma and no one to be with. I was alone, and that was the way it was going to be. That was over."

She moved back to Pennsylvania and found a government job as an administrative assistant. At night she found reassurance and self-revulsion with men she met in bars, men she felt would have her: "Losers—no job, no car, drugs, no money." And she searched online, during all the idle hours her bureaucratic job provided, through the sites that came up when she typed in "disability." There were nonprofits offering advocacy, businesses selling equipment, leagues organizing handicapped sports, groups fund-raising for Third World amputees, campaigns against land mines led by Lady Di. She read nearly every sentence, as though somewhere through the links she clicked on, somewhere in the flood of unfiltered words, would be a phrase of wisdom or a breakthrough of science that would change what was unchangeable.

Then she landed on an advertisement for models at a site

run by Carol Davis Productions. "It was the first time I'd heard of it. It was, wow, this is bizarre. Maybe years earlier it would have been, this is perverse, disgusting. But it wasn't that. I was intrigued. I didn't understand. You mean they're attracted to amputee women? And why wouldn't anyone have told me about this? None of the physical therapists. None of the surgeons or prosthetists. It was weird to me, these men, but a million things were running through my head. I was kind of happy, excited. Maybe I wouldn't have to be alone. I started checking other sites. What's the psychological part? Is this an attraction like to large breasts or blond hair? Is this the same thing? How does a person get this way? Why was this? Did something happen to them in their childhood? And I was mad. I was pissed. How could I not have known about this? Every professional I had come into contact with hadn't let me know."

She sent a message to Carol Davis, who'd lost a leg herself, and they e-mailed back and forth. Soon Laura was being photographed and videoed: playing wheelchair basketball, swimming, operating the hand controls on the van she'd learned to drive, snorkeling, parasailing, trying to monoski. She was flying around the country for the shoots and taking in sixty thousand dollars for her share of the sales.

In none of the images was she dressed in anything less than a bathing suit. The porn on sites like Davis's could look demure, even quaint—except that, for the customers, the points of craving were often on full display. Still, there seemed to be a difference between this and conventional porn. In some of the videos the models were fully clothed, their amputations covered; the images were simply of them confronting challenges. That was the attraction: Laura shooting baskets or attempting to ski.

She mentioned, to a few friends, that she'd been doing some modeling.

"What kind of modeling?"

"Disabled-woman modeling," she answered.

"For what?"

"Well, to show that we're like everybody else, that we can be accepted as who we are."

"That's good."

"That we can be accepted not just as disabled."

"That's great."

"That we can be sexual."

"Oh."

They wondered who the videos were for, and she explained that health professionals would use them for training. "But," she forced herself to add, "there are also people, mostly men, who like women with disabilities, amputees especially."

"You mean?"

"Attracted to them."

Her friends were open with their thoughts: that this was strange, that it was sick. They told her they worried about her self-esteem, worried that she was letting herself be used. One day Laura's brother, who was a UPS driver, had a package spill open on his truck. The package held magazines bound for a devotee. They didn't include any pictures of Laura, and he kept his discovery of the phenomenon to himself until one day Laura worked up her courage and asked him, as if casually, if he'd ever heard of such men. She'd never gone this far with her family. She'd never spoken about her modeling. She figured that her brother, the one she felt was the smartest of her siblings, would be the most sympathetic. He told her about the package. He told her it was revolting. With her family, that was the last time she raised the subject.

Online, in amputee chat rooms, some of the women warned that devotees were stalkers, predators. She learned, too, how specific their preferences could be, that some wanted SAEs, single arm amputees with the amputation above the elbow; that others hoped for women like Laura, DAKs, with double leg-amputations above the knee; that some liked single left-leg stumps the best; that others dreamed of perfect scars.

Sometimes she agreed with her friends, her brother. It was sick. And it was frightening. And it was infuriating to think that men could have their favorites in this way, that they could choose between calamities that had wrecked women's lives. But was a preference for a single arm really all that different from a preference for a certain color hair, a certain tone of skin or shape of face or type of body? And weren't there creeps among men of all kinds?

"A big chunk of my life, I kind of wanted to be a model. But I wasn't tall enough and all that, and it's funny how it turned out. I lost my legs, and there I was. What it did for me, it made me feel good about myself."

BEYOND the comical thoughts of secret government studies and nuclear fallout, Ron wondered about scientific reasons. There were few studies, and their science was suspect. It was safe to say that most devotees had been drawn to the disabled since childhood, since before they'd felt the attraction as palpably sexual, that most were men, that there were gays as well as straights among them. It was safe to say that some were aroused, too, by the thought of being amputees themselves, but that this desire was probably a distinct paraphilia, one that enticed and tormented a few men to the point that they carried out their longings, cutting off their legs with chain saws or contracting with surgeons—there was a willing and well-known doctor in Scotland—to perform the operations. It was clear that, like Ron, most devotees were glad to have their arms and legs, and that many, like him, were attracted to women without limbs both by visually charged lust and by emotionally infused admiration for the way the women coped. And it was clear that no one had a clue about the desire's source.

Was some sort of displaced castration fantasy involved? Or a not-so-sublimated wish to commit violence against women, to cut, to dismember, to destroy? Was there a yearning to play savior? A need for control? Ron had his own half-joking theory built on thoughts of evolution, of ancestral adaptation: his desire derived from the prehistoric savannah, where predatory animals had learned to recognize crippled prey as the easiest to catch and kill. "Am I the lion going after the lame antelope? How primitive is this? There's so much that's primal in our sexual nature. But when people say to me, 'You go after disabled women because they're easy to get,' I have to tell them, 'They're not easy to get. Trust me. They're much more reticent, very much more resistive. They've got this whole attitude: what do you want me for? And they've got this independence they've had to fight to achieve.'"

In the end, Ron didn't believe that cause could be accounted for. Rather than talk about reasons, he preferred to quote the sixteenth-century philosopher Montaigne: "It is a common proverb in Italy that he does not know Venus in her perfect sweetness who has not lain with the cripple." The legs of the lame or of the amputated, Montaigne wrote, required less bodily "nourishment" and so left more sustenance for the genitals. The vagina was more "vigorous" in crippled women.

Krafft-Ebing had given a more simple blessing. After examining and taking the history of a thirty-year-old civil servant who yearned for women with a left-footed limp, women whose deformity would match that of a girl he'd played with when he was seven, the doctor wrote: "I enlightened the patient on the subject, and told him that it was difficult, if not absolutely impossible, for medical science to obliterate a fetishism so deeply rooted by old associations, but expressed the hope that if he made a limping maid happy in wedlock, he himself would find happiness also."

But, for Ron, the words from past centuries were only somewhat more satisfying than the search for explanations. And what he wanted anyway, far more than psychology or history, was the revelation of art, a way to evoke his erotic vision in images. Then, at a Manhattan museum, he rediscovered Bellmer, whose work he'd first been staggered by in college. He confronted what the surrealist had called his "plastic anagrams," the photographs of his dismembered dolls. Ron stood before the broken doll at the base of the stairs, the doll with two pairs of legs and groins in the aftermath of passion and in the aftermath of rape. Bellmer had been fascinated by anagrams, by the connections and meanings latent within words. *Beil*, the word for ax in German, became *lieb*, the word for love, he pointed out in one of his essays. And *lieb* in turn became *leib*, the word for body. He sensed the oracular in such rearrangements, truths of the human psyche lying dormant and waiting in plain sight to be found. Through his dolls, he felt he could do the same with the body. The body parts were the letters, and their violent reordering would reinvent the body's language and unmask its messages and lead to a shaman's wisdom.

Ron wondered if he could do the same without the dolls. Until he stood facing Bellmer's photographs, his own were fairly standard portraits—flattering, sentimental—of women with disabilities. The braces and hooks and stumps gave the images an unsettling edge, but the abnormalities were treated discreetly, kept at an emotional periphery. Now a brazen impulse took hold. "I plugged into the sense of disarticulation in the dolls, the idea of plastic anagrams. If I could meet Bellmer today, I would ask why he used the dolls. Perhaps the answer is that he couldn't deal with a human being. He was exploring elements of sexuality that people can't normally handle. The dolls were symbolic. And by using dolls he could get away with making them young, putting them in that time of almost unfettered sexuality."

Bellmer seemed to have traveled far on a journey toward something primitive, and the photographs stirred, in Ron, a barely articulate erotic understanding and artistic ambition. "The elemental body" was the phrase that came to him. "There's something about making love to a legless woman—there's nothing in the way. It's a clear path, it's very primal to me." There was an artistic depth he might reach, he thought, through the bodies that held such power over him.

The first body he used belonged to a prostitute who went by the name Johnny Bardot. Until she'd been pushed in front of a subway, she'd been a madam at a high-priced bordello on the Upper East Side. Now she was turning tricks, working from a wheelchair on the streets west of Times Square. A friend of Ron's delivered her to him.

The friend, whom Ron had met through men like the Korean War pilot who had created a kind of community around their desire, was the sort of devotee who sent some amputees and their advocates into missions of warning and outbursts of rage. He traveled the world, searching for amputee women, and approached almost every one that he saw. The approaches weren't impolite; he would have seemed a harmless player, Ron thought, had his target been women with all their limbs; instead he seemed almost criminal, striking up conversations in train stations and at prosthetics conventions. He noticed Johnny Bardot one night from his car, knew right away that Ron would want to photograph her, and set up a meeting.

Ron paid her for her time. He sold the pictures on a devotee Web site and gave her the profits, several thousand dollars. What he got in return was a living version of Bellmer's dolls.

The photographs are at once visionary and political. In one—probably the most conventionally pornographic of the series—Bardot sits on an impeccably smooth gray floor. She wears a white corset that laces up the back. The stays cling to her body, which she kept in shape with a fanatical routine of modified push-ups and crunches. She looks back over one shoulder at the camera, her face framed and shadowed by her profusion of hair, which enwraps her cheekbones and chin and tumbles over her shoulders in loose curls of oak and gold. A white bow, a tribute to Bellmer, lies slightly off-center on her head, seeming to slide down the shimmering ringlets. She smiles minimally, seductively. Her lower body, the legs amputated close to the hips, is clothed in white stockings. Her back is arched; her ass, broad and round, is cocked toward the viewer and sits on the flawless gray surface. All is flawless, except for the absence of legs. Yet within the way of seeing dictated by the picture, within the aesthetic created by the gray that rises from the floor and forms, too, the backdrop of the image, so that Bardot seems to be posing in her own ethereal world—within the photograph, the absence of legs is not a flaw at all.

Curving delicately at its end and sheathed in white, the right stump, the only one visible because of the camera's angle, suggests the shape and perfection and allure of an egg— the stump is beautiful in itself. But the absence of legs also accentuates the sexual. Bardot's posture—back arched, ass cocked—provokes thoughts of her being locked to a man's lap, and the thoughts are not of strangeness; the thoughts are not repellent, not even remotely. It is easy to imagine that the experience of having her in this way would be far more primitive, more pure, more powerful than being straddled by a typical woman.

In another photograph her deconstruction is as gentle as it is violent. Sitting in an antique chair whose legs draw elegant curves, she wears an old-fashioned white undergarment. The bodice is tight, the thigh-length skirt spreads in a bloom of crinoline. She faces the camera, her features almost completely obliterated by shadow, only a sliver of nose and half of her lips illuminated in a way that speaks of sadness and keen vulnerability and a longing for the touch of an exquisite, tender lover.

It seems she has found him. She wears one prosthetic leg and extends it toward the viewer: toward that touch, that lover. A wide band of lace adorns that artificial thigh, and she offers it to the slow and tender man, the man who will, at every moment, treat her vulnerability as precious; she asks him silently to slide the lace down and off her leg.

She wants him, as well, to remove the leg itself. The other prosthetic already lies on the floor below the chair. He has taken it in his hands and taken it off and placed it aside. He has done this just as he might unlace or unbutton an article of her clothing and slip it away from her skin. Removing the first prosthetic is like the start of a deep undressing. Removing the other will be the completion. She sits within the bloom of crinoline with one leg gone and the other waiting. She asks him to go that far because he goes so softly.

Yet he is tearing her apart, tearing her limb from limb. That is the impulse lurking within his softness, and the result, no matter how slowly and gently he proceeds, is that one leg has been pulled off and the other is about to follow. This is their desire: his bringing destruction, her being destroyed, decomposing, taking on a more primal form. This is their inexorable mission as they make love.

But unlike Bellmer's images, the portraits of Bardot have a political purpose, a "usefulness" as Bellmer contemptuously put it, that accompanies the artistic vision. These are statements of enlightened outcry at the same time that they are invocations of darkness. They say: *Look* at this woman. She is an amputee, someone from whom you would avert your eyes, but she is beautiful, complex, as fully human as anyone you know. *Look. Stare. Take her in. Allow her in. Allow her to be.*

And in some of the pictures, the message is yet more bold. There is no plea to be seen, recognized, permitted her humanity. There is presumption and self-advertisement: *I am splendid by any standard, and you will look, stare, want.* For all her welcoming of destruction, the photographs proclaim a liberation, a refusal to be reduced, an exultant strength.

Johnny Bardot, whose real name was Janet, bought heroin with the money Ron paid her. She had always used. But now dependency deepened, addiction took hold, and sometimes she couldn't be photographed when they had arranged to work. She was nodding out. Always she had assumed any pose he described. She had never protested; body and being had been pliant. Now she deteriorated to the point that she couldn't perform. Willingness became vacancy. The lens couldn't find the life within her. And eventually she disappeared. But until then, she was much more than a model; she was an actress capable of embodying all the layers, all the contradictions he hoped to render. She poses, in one frame, with a pair of dark wooden crutches. She wears antiquated prosthetics that lace up along the thighs. One of the laces is loose, and part of the knee on the other leg is missing. Plainly the contraptions can't work, but their leather and laces are beautiful, and she is determined to use them. She leans forward and tries to rise out of a chair, to lever herself onto the crutches with her thick, muscled arms. Her head tilts almost coquettishly, and her oak-and-gold hair tumbles to that side, but there is nothing coquettish about her effort. She is fragile and stubborn, helpless and self-sufficient, broken and complete. She is lovely, and it is hard not to fall in love.

THE jazz club was down a set of difficult stairs, impossible with a wheelchair. The maître d' told him where to go, and he wheeled Laura down the block. At times, she didn't wear her prosthetics, though she was proficient on them—they were awkward and exhausting. He wheeled her around the corner and through the front doors of an apartment building. They rode the building's elevator down, navigated a basement corridor, entered the back door to the club's kitchen. He wheeled her between the flaming stoves and mammoth refrigerators, between the chopping and sautéing, through the swinging doors and into the club. This, if you were in a wheelchair, was the only way.

After nineteen years, Ron's marriage to Elizabeth was falling apart. "Not because we were a devotee and an amputee," he said, "but because we were a man and a woman. Our marriage failed for the same screwed-up reasons that half of all marriages do." He'd seen images of Laura on Carol Davis's Web site, and Davis had relayed his request that she model. At the start, she was, for him, simply a replacement for Johnny Bardot. And he, for her, was someone to avoid dating. Intrigued as she was by what compelled devotees, and open as she was to the idea of their desire, she had decided she didn't want to come any closer than conversation; she had told herself she didn't want to be touched by anything more than a photographer's lens. She bent her rule, she remembered, "because Ron was successful, a big-city person, intelligent, educated." Hours before their evening at the jazz club, they'd finished an all-day shoot, a session with a modern dancer, an attempt to replicate the delicate lines of Degas despite the stolid thickness of stumps and the weight of prosthetics.

The bassist Ron Carter was playing that night. Carter's girlfriend lived in Ron's small building, but even without that, the musician might have recognized him—Ron was a regular at his gigs. Carter nodded and steered his band into "Blue Monk" as Ron wheeled Laura to a table. He knew it was Ron's favorite. The bass climbed the song's staircase of notes, skipping upward and then, distracted, stopping to dance on the steps before reaching the top.

At the shoot earlier that day, Ron had been "this neurotic photographer who was driving me insane," Laura recalled. "Pacing back and forth in this loft he'd rented, pacing and yelling. He hated what the stylist was doing with my hair. He thought it was too severe. He'd never worked with her before, and he was freaking out. 'What the fuck are you doing? What the fuck are you doing?' Over and over. Chaos. The costumes wouldn't sit right. He was chain-smoking and swearing. No one could find the electrical outlets. And we were waiting for the dancer. He'd hired someone from the Dance Theater of Harlem, but at the last minute he had to go with the troupe to Washington to perform for the president, and we were waiting for his replacement. It was mayhem. Ron was not a human being."

He became one as Carter plucked his bass, performing subtle, lilting acrobatics. And afterward, with the months of phone calls and e-mails between New York and Pennsylvania, Ron's being a devotee put her off less and less. "We started to talk all the time, and I was thinking, This is so wonderful. He was the first man I could totally relate to. I didn't have to hide any of my dreams. I was thinking, This is the neatest thing in the world. I could tell he was everything I wanted, a friend and a companion and someone who accepted me totally for myself." She cut herself off as she spoke to me. "This is going to make me cry."

She sat, her voice breaking, in the living room of the house they'd bought together a year earlier, five years after they'd met. It was a few minutes' drive from downtown in a Pennsylvania city, in a community of quiet lanes and cul-de-sacs, of well-pruned shrubs and sloping lawns. The one-story house had a stone façade and a small swimming pool where, in the summer, Laura did laps to exercise her arms and "limblets"—the word she preferred to "stumps." Inside, all was sleek and modern. She sat on a square-backed couch, with her prosthetics off. Lately she had been learning to use a new pair. Their technology was more advanced; they would give her, eventually, a bit more agility. But the process would take half a year, and she swore that this was the last time she would put herself through it, no matter what improvements science offered. Her legs leaned, at the moment, against the wall in the bedroom she shared with Ron.

He rubbed her neck as her voice gave way. "When I met her, she was right on the cusp of things."

"In his eyes, I was what he was looking for. But he was what *I* was looking for. I was coming out. I was changing."

"It sounds kind of silly, but she was a bud about to bloom."

"It's true. It was like perfect timing. I wanted somebody responsible and worldly, somebody to talk to, somebody—not to take care of me but to be nurturing. And until Ron I never had a relationship like that."

"She was out there alone."

"I was striving, but I didn't have any support. I didn't have any self-esteem. Part of me knew there was something better inside me, but I didn't have anyone to help me develop it."

Now she had graduated from college and was halfway to a master's in social work. She planned to counsel the disabled. "Everything I've ever wanted to do I'm doing now. I wanted to own a house like this. I wanted to model. I wanted a college education. And I wanted to be a psychologist, and now, in a way, I'm going to be."

She worked, as part of her master's program, at a state-funded mental health center that helped patients to find the right kind of care. The center was part of a movement in the field; it was known as a "consumer organization"—the staff were or had once been mental health patients themselves. They knew what it was to be as lost as Laura when she'd overdosed on Valium and spent ten days in a psychiatric ward.

Everyone else in the squat building of small offices had their whole bodies. Yet Laura seemed by far the most stable. The unkempt director talked incessantly about the great psychologists she'd studied with, about the great athletic achievements of her adult sons, about her own "giant balls" in standing up to practitioners who refused to listen to their patients. The center's secretary, a chiseled ex-marine in a pressed polo shirt, said repeatedly, quietly, methodically, "I have a car now," as though to convince himself of his recovery from the desolation that had hold of him. Another staffer wore her hair in a rat's tail that dangled rakishly below her psychedelic skullcap. She had no top teeth and, openly lesbian, liked to flirt with Laura. "I love those photographs," she said. "My wife and I are redecorating, and I'm going to put one up, a sexy one; I'm going to blow it up big. Laura, when are you graduating? When are we celebrating? When are we going skinny-dipping? I want to touch those legs."

In her office, Laura sat at a clutterless glass desk and took calls from the desperate. On the cork board behind her she'd tacked a poster of Freud declaring, "I've changed my mind, don't tell me about your mother . . . recover!" But with her clients she had unlimited patience. She listened for an hour and a half to a paranoid schizophrenic recounting a feud with his neighbor over a woodpile. Later she visited a lockdown ward of psychotics and tried to persuade the staff to take guidance from the patients on their treatment. This was her mission: caregivers should see patients as equals. The delusional man raging about the woodpile might well know what was best for his own care. She brought all she'd been through to her work, all the times she'd been dismissed as a cripple by the people in charge of her rehabilitation, all the times she'd been unheard, invisible.

Near the poster of Freud was a photograph of Laura perched on a kitchen counter in a short red dress. "I like that picture," she said. "It's saucy." Home was decorated with large, framed portraits: of her, of Johnny Bardot. In one, Laura sits in a silvery-pink satin dress, leaning forward with an elbow on one thigh and her chin on her fist. Her half-smile hints at self-satisfaction, defiance. She spreads her prosthetic knees and pushes the satin down between them, flaunting, concealing, taunting. But the expression on her face is more powerful than the flirtation with the fabric. Eros assumes a different form than it does in the portraits of Bardot. The sensibility has shifted with the muse. Laura radiates intelligence. Self-possession emanates more than the desire to be possessed.

Laura stands, in another photograph, wearing a two-piece gown, bodice and skirt, from centuries ago. The scarlet material is trimmed in gold brocade. From her waist the skirt billows outward, broad as a spinnaker, and grazes the floor in a huge circle. It fastens in front by a series of cobalt buttons, and she is about to start closing it, but for the moment it gapes open: a vertical window, eight or ten inches wide, runs from her waist to the floor. The gold brocade lines the opening like a ceremonial decoration, a veneration of what lies within. But nothing lies within. Inside the vast regal tent of the garment is darkness.

Because of the lighting and pose, Laura's body seems to end at the belly, to have no stumps at all. The opening exposes a pure emptiness. It is unclear how she is standing, what keeps her upright. The cavern beneath the skirt is illumined just enough to suggest that she isn't wearing her prosthetics. She stands on no legs, suspended, magical.

And that magic, along with her strong jawline turned in profile, endows her with omnipotence. The cavern is at once a universe and a womb. The vertical opening is a vaginal slit, and to slip through it, to slide the body inside the scarlet walls of the tent, to wait inside while she fastens the skirt and encloses you, swallows you, would be to live out the primal fantasy of entering the vagina not only with the penis but with everything from the skull to the toes: to be ensconced, to be consumed. The photograph's viewer, not its subject, is at risk of disintegrating, coming apart, deliquescing in the lightless world he has longed for, turning to liquid in the womb. Laura, with her half-body, will remain more than intact, more than whole.

• • •

SHE wore a ring with a white gold band and a diamond in a high setting. After six years together, they were engaged to be married. They were planning a honeymoon in Italy, including Venice, where, somehow, he would help her manage the city's steeply arched bridges, its narrow and crooked stairs, its keeling pavement, its crowded alleys, its water taxis, and where, somehow, he would help her into a gondola that would take them gliding at night along the fire-lit canals.

Their lives were merged. She was his muse, who brought life to his dreams, and he had brought life to hers. They were merged "in the million ways that make up a relationship," he said in their kitchen, as they prepared a Sunday breakfast of eggs and bagels for themselves and me.

"We have all the regular things that keep people together," she added, wheeling herself around the island counter and setting the table.

"And like the cherry on the sundae is that she's a double amputee, which brings me such happiness and pleasure and joy." He spoke plainly, and she didn't wince at his words. His attraction was an accepted fact between them, one they were accustomed to acknowledging, and though she didn't smile at his praise and his gratitude, his way of saying that he felt extremely lucky to have found a woman he melded with so well and for whom he felt such desire, it wasn't hard to imagine that she did sometimes smile at such phrases. Earlier that morning I had heard their voices across the hall in their bedroom. I had woken to their laughter.

She put out butter and jelly, and he served the eggs, and we sat down to eat. They talked about the way some in the amputee community called the attraction disgusting. "If it's disgusting," Laura asked, "what are they saying about themselves?"

She mentioned an article we'd all read in a magazine for the disabled. It spoke of the ways that doctors and psychologists and physical therapists often compounded the shame of amputees by pushing them into prosthetics not so much for the sake of independence as to spare everyone else the sight of their disfigurement. The writer recounted the stay of a quadrilateral amputee in a rehabilitation center, where she was all but forced to wear purely cosmetic legs and arms, and to cover herself in loose, long-sleeved clothing.

In reply, Ron described the relief of a friend when Elizabeth, who never wore prosthetics, had been replaced in his life by Laura. And Laura talked about the different reactions she encountered during her day, depending on whether she had put on her artificial legs. Her words made me think of something else she'd once told me, that she was proud of her life and in love with Ron, but that the truth was she felt plagued by wondering if she could win a normal man. She knew that such thinking was perverse. She knew that it spoke of self-loathing, that normal was a worthless notion, that it held only the power she allowed it. She knew better, knew she should purge her longing, but couldn't help herself. She couldn't get rid of this desire.

Yet I had heard her laughter float across the hall from a master bedroom with leopard-print pillowcases and a leopard-print comforter, laughter that was light and warm, the laughter of being beloved. And then she had emerged, resplendent, wearing a man's white dress shirt, to make breakfast with her fiancé.

After we ate, they led me out from the kitchen into the garage. They showed me a contraption: two bicycles connected side by side. She didn't have the balance to ride on her own, and a typical tandem, one rider behind the other, wouldn't offer enough stability, either. He'd come across the side-by-side design in an old disability magazine, ordered the connector, and gone to a local bike shop for help in attaching it. But the device wouldn't fit with any of the shop's bicycles. Ron was about to give up when he wondered if using old-fashioned bikes might be a solution. He found a pair on eBay, and returned to the shop, where the mechanic, sympathetic to the project because his mother was blind, set to work again. And this time, all went smoothly. The contraption was perfect.

Suddenly Ron and Laura were peddling and coasting beside each other, flying through their own breeze, bound together, free.

There was only one problem. Soon he was gasping for breath. He wasn't as strong, wasn't in her kind of shape. He needed to stop, to turn around, when she wasn't at all ready, when she was barely breathing hard, when she was exhilarated. She wanted to go on and on.

Acknowledgments

This is a book of trust. To all the people who taught me with the stories of their lives—the people who fill these pages and the many more who fill my thinking—thank you for your trust and your teaching. And thank you to the scientists and therapists who gave their time so generously to educate me.

Among my sources of learning is the photography of Ron Parisi, whose story I tell in "The Devotee." His work can be found at www.ronparisi.com.

This is also a book that required a great deal of faith. For that and for all her guidance, I have long been very lucky to have Suzanne Gluck as my agent—and I am lucky to have William Morris's Sarah Ceglarski, Raffaella De Angelis, Tracy Fisher, Erin Malone, and Cathryn Summerhayes on my side.

Then there is Lee Boudreaux. When we first met, I thought, I want her for my editor. My instincts were only half right, in that I guessed only half of what a wonderful editor she would be. And Dan Halpern, along with Rachel Bressler, Alison Former, Abby Holstein, Van Luu, Michael McKenzie, Greg Mortimer, Allison Saltzman, and the sales team (whose readings, starting with Jeanette Zwart's, were so thoughtful) have made Ecco a perfect home.

Ilena Silverman, my editor at the *New York Times Magazine*, gave this book its beginning and offered crucial friendship throughout its writing.

For friendship, faith, guidance, my endless gratitude to Samantha Gillison, John Gulla, William Hogeland, Roland Kelts, George Packer, Ayesha Pande, and Elissa Wald.

For my father, so much admiration, so much love.

And then:

KSF, you are in every word.

Nancy, without you, there would be no words.

And Natalie and Miles, who changed my life, without you there wouldn't be much of anything at all.

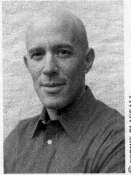

© SOPHIE BLACKALL

ABOUT THE AUTHOR

DANIEL BERGNER is a contributing writer for the *New York Times Magazine* and the author of two previous books of nonfiction—*In the Land of Magic Soldiers*, a *Los Angeles Times* Best Book of the Year and winner of an Overseas Press Club Award and a Lettre Ulysses Award for the Art of Reportage; and *God of the Rodeo*, a *New York Times* Notable Book of the Year. Bergner's writing has also appeared in *Granta, Harper's, Mother Jones, Talk*, the *New York Times Book Review*, on the op-ed page of the *New York Times*, and is included in the *Norton Reader: An Anthology of Nonfiction*. He lives in Brooklyn, New York.